Pediatric Dysphagia
Resource Guide

SINGULAR RESOURCE GUIDE SERIES

EDITOR

Ken Bleile, Ph.D.
Department of Communicative Disorders
University of Northern Iowa
Cedar Falls, Iowa

ASSOCIATE EDITORS

Brian Goldstein, Ph.D.
Communication Sciences
Temple University
Philadelphia, Pennsylvania

Sharon Glennen, Ph.D.
Department of Communication Sciences
and Disorders
Towson University
Towson, Maryland

Carole Roth, Ph.D.
Department of Speech Pathology
Hennepin County Medical Center
Minneapolis, Minnesota

Amy Weiss, Ph.D.
Department of Speech Pathology and Audiology
University of Iowa
Iowa City, Iowa

Tricia Zebrowski, Ph.D.
Department of Speech Pathology and Audiology
University of Iowa
Iowa City, Iowa

Pediatric Dysphagia
Resource Guide

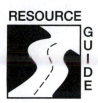

RESOURCE GUIDE

Kelly Dailey Hall, Ph.D., CCC/SLP
Northern Illinois University
DeKalb, Illinois

SINGULAR

THOMSON LEARNING™

Australia   Canada   Mexico   Singapore   Spain   United Kingdom   United States

SINGULAR

━━━━━━✦━━━━━━ ™

THOMSON LEARNING

Pediatric Dysphagia Resource Guide
by Kelly Dailey Hall, Ph.D.

Business Unit Director:
William Brottmiller

Acquisitions Editor:
Marie Linvill

Editorial Assistant:
Cara Jenkins

Executive Marketing Manager:
Dawn Gerrain

Channel Manager:
Kathryn Bamberger

Production Manager:
Barb Bullock

Production Editor:
Sandy Doyle

Library of Congress Cataloging-in-Publication Data
Hall, Kelly Dailey.
Pediatric dysphagia resource guide/Kelly Dailey Hall
p. ; cm
Includes bibliographical references and index.
ISBN 0-7693-0063-4 (alk. paper)
1. Deglutition disorders in children.
2. Ingestion disorders in children. I Title
[DNLM: 1. Deglutition Disorders—Child.
2. Deglutition Disorders—Infant. WI 250 H177r 2000]
RJ463.I54 H35 2000
618.92'31—dc21   00-058847

NOTICE TO THE READER

Publisher does not warrant or guarantee any of the products described herein or perform any independent analysis in connection with any of the product information contained herein. Publisher does not assume, and expressly disclaims, any obligation to obtain and include information other than that provided to it by the manufacturer.

The reader is expressly warned to consider and adopt all safety precautions that might be indicated by the activities herein and to avoid all potential hazards. By following the instructions contained herein, the reader willingly assumes all risks in connection with such instructions.

The Publisher makes no representation or warranties of any kind, including but not limited to, the warranties of fitness for particular purpose or merchantability, nor are any such representations implied with respect to the material set forth herein, and the publisher takes no responsibility with respect to such material. The publisher shall not be liable for any special, consequential, or exemplary damages resulting, in whole or part, from the readers' use of, or reliance upon, this material.

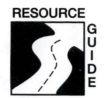

CONTENTS

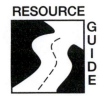

FOREWORD

The emblem for this series is a stylized road ending in an arrow. This symbol is intended to represent the goal of the series: to create books that serve as road maps to the care of communicative disorders. Like good road maps, each book gives the clinician an honest depiction of the territory, shows the various routes, and allows you the traveler to select the route best suited for your particular type of journey. Each book author is someone who knows the territory about which he or she is writing, both as a clinician and a researcher. The editorial board that advises the editors and authors is composed of some of the most respected persons in our profession. The hope of all involved in the series is that you will find the books useful and readable. Good traveling!

Ken Bleile, Ph.D.
Series Editor

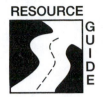

PREFACE

During the last 20 years, interest in and knowledge about swallowing disorders has increased tremendously. The majority of speech-language pathologists (SLPs) within the medical setting are routinely involved in the management of swallowing disorders in adults. In recent years, however, SLPs in both the school and hospital settings find that their caseloads include increasingly more young children with chronic feeding and swallowing problems often associated with multiple medical disorders. This change in our client population in part reflects advances in medical technology that now greatly improve the chances that medically fragile children will survive. Our caseloads in the schools are also changing because of the significant advances in federal legislation mandating that integrated services be made available to children from birth to 21 years of age (i.e., IDEA: PL 105-17). The result is that SLPs and other early intervention professionals are now involved in a broader spectrum of service delivery models and service delivery roles.

Despite the increasing number of children with complicated medical and feeding problems on our caseloads, most SLPs and other professionals working with this population did not receive training in pediatric dysphagia in their formal education. Instead, much of the training comes from continuing education efforts via workshops, state and national sponsored conferences, textbooks, journal articles, and so forth. The *Pediatric Dysphagia Resource Guide* is an effort to bring together the latest information in the assessment and treatment of pediatric feeding and swallowing disorders in an easy-to-use, clinician-friendly format. In doing so, this book has made use of a number of excellent textbooks, namely J. Arvedson and L. Brodsky's (1993) *Pediatric Swallowing and Feeding: Assessment and Management*; D. Tuchman and R. Walter's (1994) *Disorders of Feeding and Swallowing in Infants and Children: Pathophysiology, Diagnosis, and Treatment*; M. Klein and T. Delaney's (1994) *Feeding and Nutrition for the Child With Special Needs*; S. Morris and M. Klein's (1987) *Pre-Feeding Skills. A Comprehensive Resource for Feeding Development*; and L. Wolf and R. Glass's (1992) *Feeding and Swallowing Disorders in Infancy*.

The *Pediatric Dysphagia Resource Guide* is not intended as a replacement for textbooks or continuing education. Rather, it integrates existing research and information into a clinical tool in a concise, easy-to-use format. It is designed to complement existing student texts, but it will be particularly useful for the busy school or medically based clinician who needs to find information quickly.

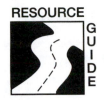

HOW TO USE THIS RESOURCE GUIDE

As our technology continues to advance, so does the opportunity for an infant's survival outside of the womb as early as 22 weeks. Many speech-language pathologists (SLPs) and occupational therapists (OTs) who are specialists in feeding and swallowing now establish oral feedings in younger and sicker children. School-based SLPs also find that their caseloads are gaining considerably more children with complex feeding and swallowing issues. To effectively intervene with the pediatric dysphagia population, the feeding specialist must have an understanding of normal infant development, medical management, the Neonatal Intensive Care Unit environment, and many other issues related to long-term management of children with feeding disorders. The *Resource Guide To Pediatric Dysphagia* provides easy access to this information, which is divided into the following sections:

❖ **Section 1: Core Knowledge.** This section provides basic information necessary for working with infants and children with feeding and swallowing problems. The information, presented in text, charts, and figures, focuses on normal infant development. Information is provided on:

- Neonatology
- Normal Developmental System Changes
- Gastrointestinal Tract
- The Role of Respiration in Swallowing
- Suck-Swallow-Breathe Sequence
- Brain Stem and Cortical Control of Deglutition
- Normal Development of Feeding Skills
- Alternate Methods of Nutritional Intake
- Overview of the Neonatal Intensive Care Unit

❖ **Section 2: Medical Disorders and Other Etiologies of Pediatric Dysphagia.** This section includes a comprehensive review of common medical disorders and treatments associated with feeding problems. Information is provided on:

- Prematurity and Respiratory Disorders
- Gastrointestinal and Gastroesophageal Track Disorders
- Central Nervous System Damage
- Peripheral Nervous System Damage
- Cardiac Defects
- Extracorporial Membraneous Oxygenation (ECMO)
- Structural Abnormalities
- Maternal Substance Abuse
- Nonorganic Failure to Thrive (FTT)

❖ **Section 3: Procedures.** This section includes charts and lists for clinical and videofluoroscopic assessment of feeding. Information is provided on:

- Assessing Prefeeding Skills
- The Clinical Feeding Evaluation
- The Videofluoroscopic Swallowing Evaluation

❖ **Section 4: Therapy for Feeding and Swallowing Problems.** This section includes charts and lists for treating infants and children with a variety of swallowing and feeding problems. Information is provided on:

- Compensatory Strategies
- Facilitative Strategies
- Transitioning From Tube to Oral Feedings

❖ **Section 5: Case Studies.** This section profiles infants and children with common feeding/swallowing problems and provides guidelines for assessment, intervention, and goal writing. Information is provided on children grouped in the following categories:

- Respiratory Compromise
- Cardiac Defects
- Gastroesophageal Problems
- Neurologic Disorders
- Behavioral Feeding Problems

❖ **Section 6: Glossary.** This section includes terms and definitions relevant to the medical aspects of pediatric dysphagia.

❖ **Section 7: Resources.** This section highlights important resources, phone numbers, addresses, Internet sites, and feeding equipment.

❖ **Section 8: References.** This section provides a bibliography relevant to pediatric dysphagia.

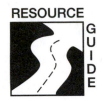

ACKNOWLEDGMENTS

This book has profited from the help and encouragement of a number of people who made the project an enjoyable experience and who rescued me from errors and infelicities of many kinds. I must begin by expressing my sincere thanks to Sadanand Singh, Marie Linvill, Ken Bleile, and the staff at Singular Thomson Learning for their limitless patience and their determination to see the book come to fruition. I am grateful to Thomas D. Dailey, the graphic line artist who furnished the illustrations for the book, for responding swiftly and efficiently to my requests for assistance. I owe a profound debt to my fellow faculty in the Department of Communicative Disorders at Northern Illinois University, especially my chair Earl "Gip" Seaver, for supporting my efforts and for affirming my conviction that I could never have found a better department to work in. This book is also informed by my personal and professional interactions with superb clinicians such as Rona Alexander, Robert Beecher, Judy Michels Jelm, and Marjorie Palmer. I give special thanks to my "best friend" and buddy for giving me more than just editorial assistance. I thank the many children and families I have known with pediatric dysphagia, who gave me the best education possible on this subject and who are the reason I wrote this resource guide. And I owe the most to my children—Hannah and Lauren—who get to have Mommy back now.

SECTION

CORE KNOWLEDGE

· ·

SETTING THE STAGE

American Speech-Language-Hearing Association's Scope of Practice Guidelines

Recognizing that many speech-language pathologists (SLPs) are involved in the diagnosis and treatment of pediatric and adult dysphagia, the American Speech-Language-Hearing Association's (ASHA's) Task Force on Dysphagia developed a statement outlining the knowledge and skills needed to provide these services (American Speech-Language Hearing Association, 2000). In general, SLPs working with infants, children, or adults with dysphagia must be competent in the following areas:

❖ Identifying persons at risk for dysphagia

❖ Conducting and interpreting clinical assessments of oral-pharyngeal and respiratory functions related to feeding

❖ Conducting and interpreting instrument-based evaluation of swallowing

❖ Developing intervention strategies (i.e., safe feeding recommendations, swallowing precautions, and therapeutic interventions)

❖ Documenting care and discharge planning

❖ Providing education, counseling, and training to patients and all other relevant individuals (i.e., family, health professionals, etc.)

Although this list is not complete, it provides an overview of the responsibilities and proficiencies needed to provide services to the dysphagia population.

NEONATOLOGY

Embryologic and Fetal Development of Feeding/Swallowing

The successful development of a fetus depends on a number of factors, both genetic and environmental. For some infants, the complex progression from fertilization to birth is besieged with countless chances for errors that result in birth defects or premature delivery that, in turn, can affect feeding/swallowing. Because of the advances in ultrasoundography, many medical conditions that contribute to dysphagia (i.e., vascular anomalies, cleft lip, upper airway anomalies, some genetic syndromes) may be detected in utero. Also, with advances in medical technology that can save very premature infants, the feeding specialist needs to have an understanding of normal embryologic and fetal development, particularly as it relates to the structures and function for development of feeding and swallowing skills.

Between weeks 3 and 8 after fertilization, the embryo develops all major systems. Initially, the embryo consists of three germ layers from which all tissues and structures of the body form. Six branchial arches (see Table 1–1) ultimately give rise to the muscles, cranial nerves, and skeleton that become the anatomic structures of speech and swallowing. Children born with arch defects often have malformations of the head and neck that affect swallowing (Moore, 1988). These include hemifacial microsomia, hypoplasia of the facial musculature, cleft lip and/or palate, and cardiac anomalies that lead to respiratory compromise associated with feeding (Jones, 1997). Treacher Collins syndrome and Pierre Robin sequence are two of the more common conditions resulting from first and second branchial arch abnormalities (Arvedson, Rogers, & Brodsky, 1993). Defects occurring during the embryologic period of development can be so well identified that physicians can pinpoint at what week (or day) the defect occurred. Table 1–2 illustrates the development of the head and neck, central nervous system, cardiac system, and respiratory system during the embryonic and fetal period.

Primitive Reflexes

The newborn infant manages her or his new existence outside of the uterus armed with protective and adaptive reflexes. Most of these reflexes are specifically designed to assist the infant in finding and safely obtaining oral nutrition. That is, they either help the infant locate food or protect the airway when swallowing. The elicitation of these reflexes is through tactile input. Newborn infants can express their rejection, tolerance, or acceptance of tactile stimulation through a variety of behavioral responses. The acceptance of tactile stimulation to the face and mouth are precursors to successful feeding and survival (Wolf & Glass, 1992). The presence or absence of specific reflexes can be indicative of the child's neurologic stability. Table 1–3 lists each of the primitive reflexes important in normal feeding/swallowing development, how to elicit the reflex, what cranial nerve is responsible for the reflex, at what age

TABLE 1–1. The Branchial Arches

Branchial Arch	Muscles	Nerves	Skeleton
1st Mandibular	Muscles of mastication (temporal, masseter, and pterygoids) mylohyoid, anterior digastric, tensor veli palatini, tensor tympani	V Trigeminal nerve, all three divisions: sensory Mandibular division: motor	Facial bones, incus, malleus, anterior ligament of malleus
2nd Hyoid	Muscles of facial expression, posterior digastric, stylohyoid, stapedius Levator veli palatini	VII Facial nerve Motor to facial muscles; sensory to anterior two thirds of tongue	Stapes, styloid process, stylohyoid ligament, lesser horn and upper part of hyoid body
3rd	Stylopharyngeus Upper pharyngeal muscles	IX Glossopharyngeal nerve Motor to pharyngeal muscles sensory; to posterior on third of tongue	Greater horn and lower part of hyoid body
4th	Pharyngeal constrictors Cricothyroid and laryngeal muscles Palatoglossus	X Vagus nerve	Thyroid and laryngeal cartilages
5th	Same as 4th branchial arch		Lower part of thyroid cartilage and laryngeal cartilages
6th	Laryngeal muscles except cricothyroid, striated muscles of esophagus	X Vagus nerve	Cricoid cartilage (probably) Arytenoid cartilages

TABLE 1–2. Development of Major Systems in the Embryo

Week 3

Head and Neck

- Nasal pactodes appear
- Primitive mouth present

Central Nervous System

- Neural plate (origin of CNS) forms neural folds then neural tube. The neural tube gives rise to:

    forebrain: cerebral hemispheres

    midbrain: adult midbrain

    hindbrain: brain stem structures

Cardiovascular System

- First functioning system
- Heart begins to circulate blood at 21–22 days

Weeks 4–8

Head and Neck

- Six branchial arches form anatomic structures of swallowing
- Eyes move medially and external ears ascend (week 5)
- Arytenoids and epiglottis begin to develop (week 5)
- Fusion of the maxillary and medial nasa processes, which forms the primary palate separating the oral and nasal cavities (week 6)
- Oronasal membrane ruptures, which forms the choana (week 6)
- Tongue begins to develop (weeks 7–8)

Central Nervous System

- Brain enlarges, 12 cranial nerves present (weeks 5–6)
- Normal brain waves can be detected, spontaneous movement (week 8)

Digestive System

- Endoderm of primitive gut forms the foregut, midgut, and hindgut (week 4)
- Vagally innervated esophagus reaches its final relative length (week 7)

Cardiovascular System

- critical period of heart development (20–50 days)
- Four chambers of heart are present (week 7)

Respiratory System

- Laryngotracheal tube develops, from which the closed larynx develops at the cranial end (week 5)
- Lung buds develop (week 6)
- Separation of the laryngotracheal tube to form larynx, trachea and lungs (ventral), and esophagus (dorsal) (weeks 5–8)

Weeks 9–12 (Fetal Period Begins)

- Head makes up one half the length of the fetus
- Facial features, limbs, hands, feet, fingers, and toes present
- CNS is functioning
- Hard/soft palate fusion (week 12)
- Fusion between nasal septum and palatine process (week 12)

Weeks 13–16

- Body length doubles
- Sex organs form
- Ossification of skeleton
- Eyes/ears move closer to final position
- Pharyngeal swallow begins

Weeks 17–20

- Pharyngeal swallow strengthens
- Fetus swallows and digests up to 50% amniotic fluid
- Suckling begins

Weeks 21–25

- With special equipment and intensive intervention, fetus may survive outside of uterus
- Substantial weight gain
- Skin becomes opaque
- Upper and lower respiratory development
- Lungs produce surfactant (week 24)

Weeks 26–29

- Primitive reflexes begin (i.e., gag, phasic bite)
- Lungs may be capable of breathing air with difficulty
- CNS maturing to improve rhythmic breathing and control body temperature

Weeks 30–33

- Head growth slows, body lengthens
- Skin becomes thicker
- "Breathing" patterns continue
- Premature infant is still unable to safely coordinate suck, swallow, breathe

Weeks 34–36

- Premature infants may begin breast or bottle feeding
- Most infants can sustain nutrition orally

Week 37–40

- Normal gestation is 38 weeks from fertilization or 40 weeks from last menses
- Baby body fat at birth equals 16% of total body weight
- Average weight is 7 pounds
- Average length is 19 inches

to expect the reflex to begin and end, and the significance of the reflex for swallowing. Table 1–4 presents the reflexes that are important for self-feeding.

Infant Stages of Alertness and Stress Cues

Als and Brazelton (1981) recognize that full-term infants have highly organized and protective responses to manage or shut out environmental stimulation. Assessing overall state will let the feeding specialist know how the infant is adapting to and tol-

TABLE 1–3. Primitive Reflexes Related to Swallowing

Reflex	Stimulus	Behavior	Cranial Nerve(s) Involved	Present at	Diminishes by	Significance
Gag	Touch to posterior tongue or pharynx	Mouth opening, head extension and floor of mouth opening	IX (Glossopharyngeal) X (Vagus) Cortex	26–27 weeks gestation	Continues through adulthood	May or may not be related to swallowing ability. Hyper- or hyporesponse may indicate neurological problem.
Phasic Bite	Touch/stimulation to the gums	Rhythmic up and down jaw movement	V (Trigeminal)	28 weeks gestation	9–12 months of age	Precursor to mastication
Transverse Tongue Reflex	Stroking lateral surfaces of the tongue	Tongue moves toward side of stimulation	XII (Hypoglossal)	28 weeks gestation	6 months of age	Precursor to lateralization
Tongue Protrusion	Touch to anterior tongue	Tongue protrudes from mouth	XII (Hypoglossal)	38–40 weeks gestation	6 months of age	To prepare infant to eat. Important to diminish to introduce spoon feeding.
Rooting	Stroking infant's cheek/mouth	Infant turns head toward stimulation	V (Trigeminal) VII (Facial) XI (Accessory) XII (Hypoglossal)	32 weeks gestation	3 months of age	May be present longer in breast-fed infants
Suckling	Place nipple in mouth, stroke tongue or touch to hard palate	Backward and forward tongue movement and up and down jaw movement	V (Trigeminal) VII (Facial) IX (Glossopharyngeal) XII (Hypoglossal)	18 weeks gestation	6–12 months of age	Movement should be rhythmical. Two types: Nutritive-nutritional intake and nonnutritive-oral gratification.
Sucking	Same as suckling	Up and down tongue movement Smaller vertical jaw excursion Jaw moves more independently	V (Trigeminal) VII (Facial) IX (Glossopharyngeal) XII (Hypoglossal)	6–9 months of age	24 months or older	Movement should be rhythmical. Lip seal around nipple is firmer.

TABLE 1–4. Reflexes That May Influence Development of Self-Feeding Skills

Reflex	Stimulus	Behavior	Present at	Diminishes by	Significance
Grasp	Place index finger in infant's palm. Gently press.	Infant grasps finger	Birth to 2 months of age	4–6 months of age	For finger feeding and holding cup, spoon, and bottle
Babkin	Apply deep pressure to infant's palm	Infant opens mouth, closes eyes, and brings head forward	Birth	3 months of age	To bring hand to mouth. Receive food into oral cavity
Palomental	Touch infant's palm	Infant's chin wrinkles	Birth	3 months of age	To bring hand to mouth
Startle	Sudden movement backward or presentation of loud noise	Extension and abduction of arms and legs	Birth	3 months of age	Persistence interferes with infant's ability to bring hands to mouth
Asymmetrical Tonic Neck (ATNR)	Turn infant's head to one side	Face-side arm and leg extend. Skull-side arm and leg flex.	Birth to 4 months of age	4–6 months of age	Also known as "fencer's" position. Persistence affects infant's ability to bring hands to midline and to grasp and regard object at the same time.
Moro	Sudden head drop backwards	Abduction of arms with extension of elbows, wrist, and fingers followed by subsequent adduction of arms with shoulders and flexion of elbows	28 weeks gestation	5–6 months of age	To "break up" predominant flexion postures at birth. Persistence may delay acquisition of head control.

Source: Adapted from Morris and Klein (1987).

erating her or his environment and readiness to feed. Evaluating infant stages of alertness as presented in Table 1–5 is particularly important when working with medically fragile or neurologically immature infants. Each infant is an individual and therefore there is no specific "ideal" stage for feeding all infants. Some infants begin feedings best at Stage 3, whereas others are most successful when feedings are initiated at Stage 4. It is important to note the infant's state before, during, and after feedings and determine which state is optimal for feeding (Wolf & Glass, 1992).

These stages of alertness are also helpful when working with the preterm infant. The premature infant is often very sick and unaccustomed to the Neonatal Intensive Care Unit (NICU) environment where lights, sounds, and tactile stimulation are grossly different from the environment of the uterus. Historically, there have been many studies showing the detrimental effects of the premature infants' constant exposure to light (Fielder, 1993; Messner, 1978), noise (American Academy of Pediatrics, Committee on Environmental Noise, 1997; Anagnostaki, 1980; Blennow, Svenningsen, & Almquist, 1974; Long, Philip, & Lucey, 1980a), and handling (Long, Philip, & Lucey, 1980b).

Driven by the hypothesis that premature infants experience a contrast between what their immature nervous systems are expecting and what the world outside of the uterus is presenting, we now believe that premature infants learn to adapt to the stresses in their environment through the interaction of physiologic, motor, and behavioral processes. This interaction is referred to as "synaction." The synactic model of physiologic stability is the foundation on which motor and behavioral organization occur normally in full-term infants (Als, 1982). Preterm infants, however, have difficulty establishing stability and subsequently have difficulty establishing self-regulation and modulation. They are particularly susceptible to attentional disorganization and therefore require support from their environment to help them self-regulate and function effectively (Als & Gilkerson, 1995).

The caregiver feeding a high-risk infant can use this synactic model to observe signs that the infant gives to indicate levels of stress and tolerance of the feeding. These signs, adapted from the work of Als (1982, 1986), can be grouped into three systems: Attention-Interaction System, Motor System, and Autonomic System (see Table 1–6). Successful feeding of the premature infant depends on (a) her or his ability to attain and maintain an appropriate state of alertness for feeding and (b) the caregiver's ability to monitor infant stress cues so that changes in the environment can be made to facilitate feeding.

NORMAL DEVELOPMENTAL SYSTEM CHANGES

Anatomy-Maturational Considerations

Newborn infants with intact anatomy and neurologic function most often quickly become efficient feeders. Compared to an older child, their oral and pharyngeal cavities are smaller. Because of the relatively small mandible and fat pads in the cheeks, the tongue fills the oral cavity and seems specifically designed to hold a nipple in place for feeding. The pharynx and larynx are elevated in the neck and make it anatomically difficult, although not impossible, for aspiration to occur. With age, the primary anatomical structures for swallowing shift back and downward toward an elongating pharynx.

TABLE 1–5. Infant Stages of Alertness

Stage 1 (Deep Sleep)

- Sleeping infant with regular respiratory patterns
- No rapid eye movements (REMs)
- No spontaneous movements of limbs (but *may* "startle" or jerk)
- Slow response to deep external stimulation

Stage 2 (Light Sleep)

- Sleeping infant with regular and irregular respiratory patterns
- REMs are apparent, eyes may appear half-closed
- Spontaneous movements of limbs that are random
- Sucking movements seen

Stage 3 (Dozing/Drowsy)

- Eyes open but the infant does not appear awake *or*
- Eyes flutter open/closed
- Infant shifts positions, regular movements of the limbs
- Infant responds easily to stimulation

Stage 4 (Quiet Alert)

- Infant fully awake and focusing sustained toward a stimulus (face, sound, etc.)
- Minimal movements
- Infant slowly redirects attention to new stimulus

Stage 5 (Active Alert)

- Infant fully awake and active
- Full movements of limbs
- Eyes shift from object to object
- More vocalizations, moving toward "fussy" cries

Stage 6 (Alert Agitated)

- Infant awake and fussy
- Leg extensions, side-to-side head movements
- Irregular respirations, whimpering
- Crying (low stress level), easily comforted

Stage 7 (Crying)

- Intense crying
- Facial color changes (red)
- Limbs may exhibit tremor-like shaking
- Difficulty comforting

Source: Adapted from Brazelton (1984).

TABLE 1–6. Evaluation of Infant Responses to Environmental Stress

Level 1: Attention-Interaction System

If the baby demonstrates
- eye-floating
- gaze aversion
- weak cry
- staring
- glassy-eyed
- panicked, worried, or dull look

Level 2: Motor System

or
- fluctuating tone from normal to flaccid (trunk, face, extremities)
- hypertonicity (leg extensions, arching, finger splays, tongue extensions, fisting)
- excessive, diffuse movements

Level 3: Autonomic System

or
- irregular breathing
- tachypnea
- any color change such as
  - peri-oral or peri-orbital duskiness
  - mottled
  - cyanotic
  - grey
  - flushed
  - ruddy
  - paling around nostrils
- hiccups
- spitting up
- sneezing
- sigh
- yawning
- seizures
- grunting
- tremors
- startles

try
- giving the infant a "time out"
- modifying the environment (reduce lights, noise, people, stimulation)
- change position/use blanket rolls for support
- swaddle/contain limbs
- provide support to hands/feet
- use slow, gentle movements
- offer one mode of stimulation at a time

Do's

1. Shield the isolette so you can detect subtle color changes.
2. Shield the infant's eyes before bringing him/her out of the isolette to feed.
3. Encourage hands near mouth when feeding.
4. Handle the infant slowly and gently.
5. Help the infant wake slowly, avoid startling her/him.
6. Place infant on her/his side with arms/legs flexed after feeding. Use blanket rolls to inhibit movement.

Don'ts

1. Bump, tap, or bang the isolette as a writing surface.
2. Place anything on top of the isolette (e.g., chart) or use the isolette as a writing surface.
3. Allow the infant's legs or arms to flail when moving her/him.
4. Place the infant prone after feeding.
5. Try to feed the baby until she/he is calm and stable.

Source: Adapted from Als (1982, 1886) and Brazelton (1984).

Treatment of pediatric dysphagia is particularly challenging because of the dynamic anatomical changes that take place in the growing infant's first years of life. This section provides a review of the anatomical structures of feeding/swallowing and shows changes across time. Figures 1–1 through 1–7 illustrate the definitions presented in Appendix A (see p. 211) of each of the anatomic structures of the oral cavity, pharynx, larynx, and esophagus. Table 1–7 defines the changes with age, illustrated in Figures 1–8 and 1–9.

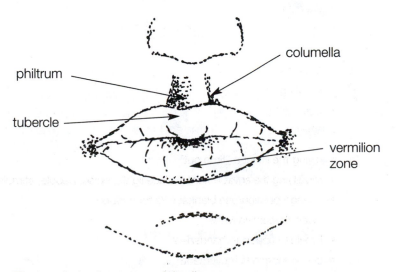

Figure 1–1. Anatomy of the lips.

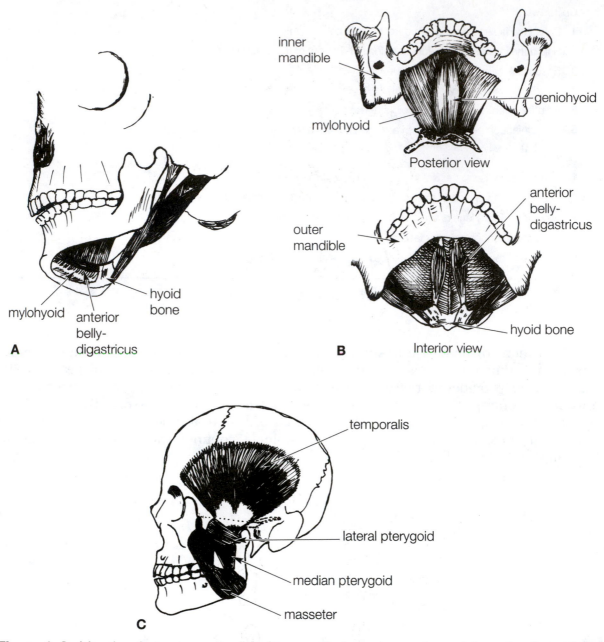

Figure 1–2. Muscles that are responsible for mandibular movements and form the floor of the mouth: **A.** A schematic showing the relationship among the mylohyoid muscle, digastricus muscle, and hyoid bone. **B.** A schematic showing posterior and interior views of the floor of the mouth. **C.** A schematic showing the relationship among the temporalis, pterygoid, and masseter muscles. (Views adapted from Seikel et al. [2000].)

Motor Development Underlying Feeding/Swallowing

From birth on, a child must adapt to a changing environment. Through brain development and learning experiences, children begin to take control of their world. Motor development is the primary basis on which children learn to adapt, interact, and

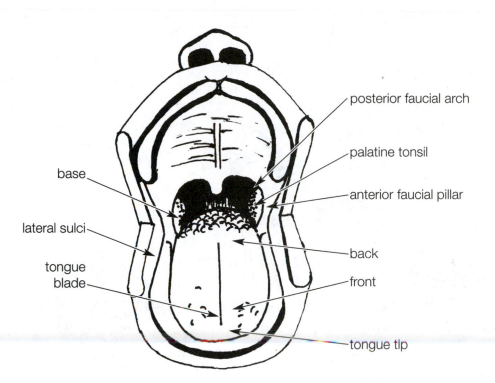

Figure 1–3. Anatomy of the oral cavity of an infant. (Adapted from Crelin [1987].)

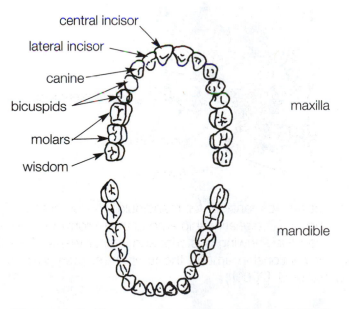

Figure 1–4. Permanent teeth. (After Zemlin [1988].)

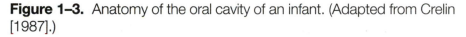

manage their environment. Motor development progresses from "head to toe," that is, first children gain head control before they sit, crawl, stand, and eventually walk. There is also a natural order of motoric events that are precursors to the following

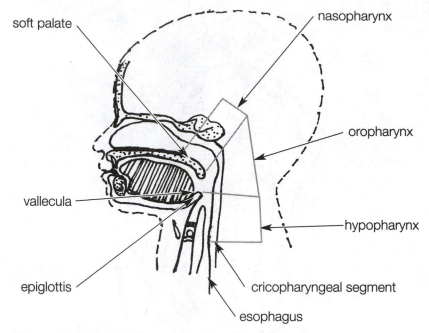

Figure 1–5. Midsagittal drawing of the oral and pharyngeal cavities of an infant.

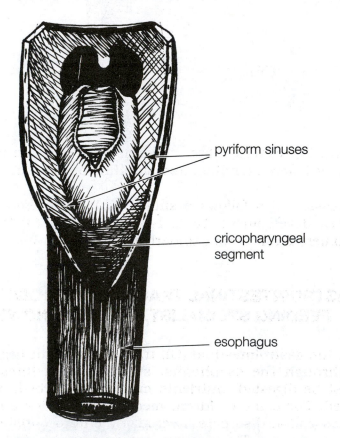

Figure 1–6. Posterior view of the oral and pharyngeal cavities of an infant.

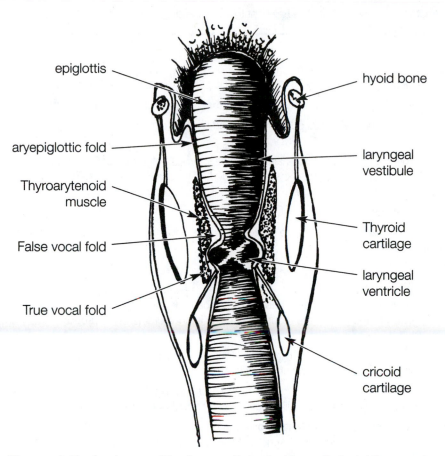

Figure 1–7. Anatomy of the larynx. (Adapted from Seikel, King, and Drumright [2000].)

stages of movement. For example, first children roll over from back to front before they begin sitting, sit before standing, and stand before walking (Batshaw & Perret, 1998).

Feeding progression also follows a similar order of events that are intricately connected to motoric development. Table 1–8 summarizes the important motor and oral-motor developmental milestones underlying feeding/swallowing.

GASTROINTESTINAL TRACT: WHAT DOES THE FEEDING SPECIALIST NEED TO KNOW?

Even before birth, the gastrointestinal (GI) tract of an infant begins its lifelong duty of moving food through the esophagus, stomach, and intestines. During this process, food must be digested, nutrients must be absorbed, and waste products must be eliminated. For some children, medical conditions affecting the GI tract (e.g., reflux, malabsorption disorders, necrotizing enterocolitis) can spark the start of chronic feeding challenges. This section summarizes the anatomy and physiology of normal GI functioning, and Section 2 presents GI tract disorders in infancy.

TABLE 1–7. Anatomic Changes With Age Relevant to Infant Feeding/Swallowing

Skull

- In a newborn, the facial portion of the skull constitutes approximately one eighth of the entire skull (compared to adults where the face constitutes one half of the skull). The skull is primarily made up of the cranium.
- The growth of the skull during infancy is slower than the other major divisions of the skeleton.
- The growth of the cranium almost triples during infancy and early toddler age, the rate of growth slows down by age 7, and at age 10 the brain reaches 90% of it's volume.
- Facial growth after age 1 is markedly faster than the cranium. Growth of the lower facial part of the skull is caused by the lateral expansion of the hard palate and the development of the maxillary sinuses. The face vertically elongates over time, and the oral/oropharynx enlarge.
- At 2 years the orbits increase to half their postnatal growth.
- Postnatal growth of the lower facial part of the skull is caused by the lateral expansion of the hard palate and the development of the maxillary sinuses.

Oral Cavity and Tongue

- In a newborn, the tongue fills the oral cavity and is solely located in the oral cavity. The tongue makes contact with the gums laterally and with the roof of the mouth above. An infant's oral cavity is proportionately smaller to the skull compared to an adult.
- Between 2 and 4 years, the posterior one third of the tongue starts it's descent into the pharynx. The tongue moves posteriorly and inferiorly. This descent is completed by 9 years of age.
- At birth, the hard palate is short (2.3 cm long) and broad and only slightly arched. The palate contains five to six folds that will be broken down into mound-like elevations by adulthood. The folds aid in suckling for nipple hold.
- The soft palate grows in length and thickness most markedly starting from 18 months to 24 months. The increase in length levels off at 4–5 years, and the thickening of the palate levels off at 14–16 years of age.

Fat Pads

- Adipose tissue is located in the masseter muscle. This tissue fills the lateral sulci, thus reducing the size of the oral cavity. This tissue provides sucking stability.
- The proportion of tissue reduces over time.

Mandible

- In a newborn, the halves of the mandible are not fused and joined by a fibrous tissue at the mandibular suture. At birth, rami are short and broad and sit at a 140° angle to the body. The body is longer than the rami.
- At birth, the mandible is relatively smaller so that the oral cavity size is reduced.
- At the end of the first year and the beginning of the second year, the halves fuse.
- Into adulthood, the rami will become more angled at 110–120°, and the body of the mandible and the rami will be equal in length.

Larynx

- At birth, the newborn infant's larynx is short (about 2.0 cm in length), one third that of an adult.
- The epiglottis is larger and is in direct contact with the soft palate.
- The pyriform sinuses are elevated and smaller in infants.
- At birth, the space between the hyoid bone and the thyroid cartilage is small, if there is any space at all.
- At birth, the larynx and hyoid bone are both elevated when the infant is eating, facilitating nasal breathing.
- As the tongue descends at ages 2–4, so does the larynx. The larynx descends from C3 or C4 to C6 by age 5, eventually arriving at C7 in adulthood.

Pharynx

- At birth, the nasal portion of the pharynx is a narrow tube that curves gradually down to join the oral part of the pharynx, lacking definition.
- At 5 years of age, the posterior wall of the nasal portion of the pharynx and the oral portion of the pharynx intersect at an oblique angle, and eventually during puberty will form a 90° angle.
- After the posterior one third of the tongue descends (between 2–4 years), the tongue makes up part of the anterior wall of the pharynx

Trachea

- At birth, the trachea is at C6 and remains there throughout adulthood.
- In an infant, the trachea tilts on a diagonal posteriorly. In toddlers, the trachea is more vertically oriented.

Esophagus

- At birth, the esophagus begins at C4 to C6 and ends at C9. In an adult, the starting and ending of the esophagus begins one to two vertebra higher.

Skeletal Vertebrae

- At birth, the average length from the 1st cervical vertebra to the fifth lumbar vertebra is 19–20 cm (40% of the total length). No fixed curves are present.
- A flexible cervical curve appears when the infant can raise her/his head.
- A flexible lumbar curve appears between 1 and 2 years, when the child starts to walk.
- The second cervical vertebra (the axis) consists of four ossification centers. The four centers fuse into a single bone between the third and sixth years.

Source: Compiled from Crelin, E. (1987). *The human vocal tract*. New York: Vantage Press.

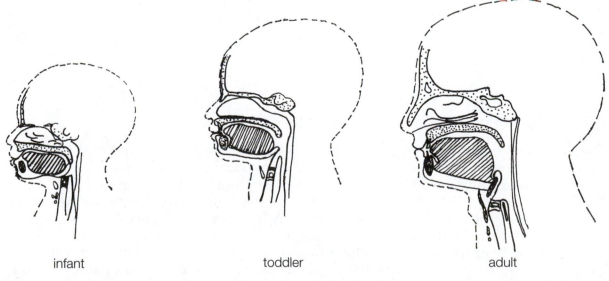

infant   toddler   adult

Figure 1–8. Drawing of an infant, toddler, and adult showing the changes in the relationship among anatomical structures with age.

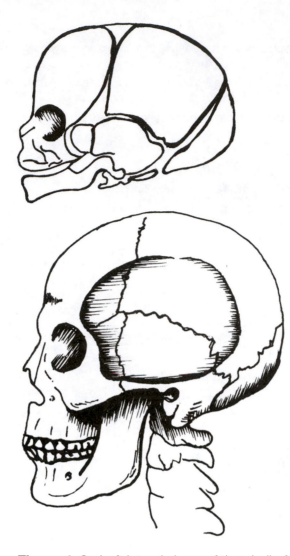

Figure 1–9. Left lateral views of the skull of a human full-term newborn infant and an adult. Comparison of an infant and an adult. (Adapted from Crelin [1987].)

Anatomy and Physiology of the GI Tract

The process of deglutition begins when the food enters the oral cavity and is manipulated and processed to a bolus ready to swallow. Food travels to the stomach through primary and secondary peristalsis of the esophagus. The anatomical capacity of a newborn's stomach is 30–35 millileters (ml). This increases to 100 ml at the end of the first month (Crelin, 1973). Once in the stomach, acids and other fluids partially digest the food, which then continues to the duodenum (see Figure 1–10). The upper parts of the small intestine (duodenum, jejunum) receive pancreatic juice (e.g., enzymes, water, electrolytes) and bile acids from the common bile duct to further break down and simplify the food into sugars, lactose, proteins, and so forth. The lower part (ileum) absorbs nutrients and passes waste to the large intestine and

TABLE 1–8. Developmental Motor Milestones

Months	Developmental Motor Milestones	Motoric Development Underlying Feeding	Developmental Milestones of the Jaw	Developmental Milestones of the Tongue	Developmental Milestones of the Lips/Cheeks
Birth–1	• reflexive movement of limbs • lifts head while on stomach, but cannot support head when held upright	• sucks on finger put near infant's mouth	• phasic bite • minimal control of gradation	• thinly contoured tongue • tongue and jaw work in unison • restricted movement due to large size compared to other structures • gag	• pads of fatty tissue surrounded by cheek muscle that is not used • pursed for suckling/sucking • due to mechanical movement of jaw, lips make contact • rooting
1–2	• moves arms smoothly in a circle • swipes at objects • holds head up briefly while on stomach • raises head while sitting supported but head bobs	• able to bring hands to mouth when lying down or sitting up	• phasic bite persists • movement same as newborn	• extension and retraction during suck(l)ing • tongue remains in mouth at rest, may protrude past gums when swallowing	• rooting strong • although some separation may be noted, lips typically move in unison with other facial structures
3–5	• 3 months: voluntary body control. Lifts head and chest while prone. Holds head up with minimum bobbing while sitting supported. Reaches and grasps. Keeps hands open frequently. • 4 months: Head turns in all directions whether prone or seated. Head normally held at midline and aligned with trunk when sitting supported. Reach is inaccurate. Grasps small objects put into hand. Brings objects to mouth.	• baby is beginning to sit up • gaining head, trunk control • able to bring hand to mouth while object is in hand	• phasic bite diminishing • improved head control possibly affects stabilization of jaw	• relaxed appearance • separation of movement within the front, mid, and back of tongue • protrudes tongue while swallowing • gag elicited on half to one third back of tongue • 5 months: inhibition of tongue movement increased	• rooting diminishes • reduction of sucking pads • development of facial muscles • control of central portion of lips • separation of lip movements • refinement of lower lip stability and upper lip activity • increased lip and cheek activity while suckling/sucking

(continued)

TABLE 1–8. (continued)

Months	Developmental Motor Milestones	Motoric Development Underlying Feeding	Developmental Milestones of the Jaw	Developmental Milestones of the Tongue	Developmental Milestones of the Lips/Cheeks
3–5	• *5 months:* Sits supported for up to 30 minutes. Rolls from stomach to back. Can be easily pulled to stand. Swaps objects from hand to hand.				
6–9	• *6 months:* Shoulder and head more stable. Turns head freely. Sits straight slightly supported or in a chair. Balances well. Reaches with one arm, grasps, and brings to mouth. Turns and twists in all directions. Creeps. • *7 months:* Holds without palm. Transfers objects from hand to hand. Cuts first tooth. Pushes up on hands and knees, rocks. • *8 months:* Manipulates objects to explore. Pulls up to stand but needs help to get down. Crawls. • *9 months:* Stands alone briefly. Gets down alone. Cruises. Sits unsupported. Gets into and out of sitting position alone. Explores with index finger.	• trunk stability allows for independent jaw, tongue movements • independent sitting • pincer grasp • extended reach • holds bottle • removes and replaces bottle	• phasic bite extinguished • jaw becomes more stabilized allowing for movement in smaller ranges • lateral with slight diagonal movement of jaw	• variety of actions emerging • may flatten, spread, groove tongue • up/down movement during munching • gag diminished in strength • tongue sensitive enough to detect which foods can or cannot be mashed • *8–9 months:* child able to lateralize food	• rooting extinguished • *6 months:* upper or lower lip draws in slightly and may see cheeks tighten • *6 months:* if child loses liquid, only at beginning or end of feeding • lower lip becomes active stabilizer • active use of lip corners and musculature around lips • able to keep bolus in between molars with the help of the lips and cheeks

20

Months	Developmental Motor Milestones	Motoric Development Underlying Feeding	Developmental Milestones of the Jaw	Developmental Milestones of the Tongue	Developmental Milestones of the Lips/Cheeks
10–12	• *10 months:* Crawls with bilateral leg-arm opposition. Sits from standing position. More fine control of hand movements. • *11 months:* Stands alone. Gets up from all-fours position by pushing up. Climbs up stairs. • *12 months:* Stands alone. Pushes to stand from squat. Climbs up and down stairs. Uses a crayon. Releases objects willfully. Takes first steps with support.	• fine motor skills develop	• emerging sustained controlled pressure on softer foods • controlled opening/closing (improving jaw grading ability) • may see early emergence of circular rotary action as precision and control of jaw movements improve	• uses all muscles to shape tongue • emergence of all ranges of angles of movement • improved precision, combinations, and consistency of movement patterns	• both upper and lower lips may draw in independently • active use of lips and cheeks on solids • lower lip draws in to be cleaned by upper incisors or gums • child no longer pockets food and rarely loses food • drooling is rare
13–24	• *15 months:* unceasing activity. Walks with rapid run-like gait. Walks a few steps backward and sideways. Carries objects in both hands or waves while walking. Throws ball with elbow extension. Takes off shoes and socks. Scribbles lines. • *18 months:* Walks up stairs with help. Walks smoothly, runs stiffly. Throws ball with whole arm. Throws and catches without falling. Jumps with both feet off floor. Scribbles in circles. Has muscle control for toilet training.		• *12–14 months:* will see emerging circular/rotary movement • *18–24 months:* will not need to turn head in direction of bite due to improved jaw grading skills	• child learns to swallow with tongue tip elevation and stabilization at alveolar ridge • food texture will influence tongue movement patterns • tongue moves side to side across midline • tongue becomes the major cleaner for inside mouth • *12–24 months:* jaw and tongue movements are independent of each other • *18–20 months:* child may clean lips with tongue	• continuation of sustained control of lip pressure and lip movements while tongue and jaw are moving (separation of control) • corners of lips may draw in to help control placement and assist with movement

(continued)

21

Months	Developmental Motor Milestones	Motoric Development Underlying Feeding	Developmental Milestones of the Jaw	Developmental Milestones of the Tongue	Developmental Milestones of the Lips/Cheeks
13–24	• *21 months*: Walks up and down stairs with help of railing or hand. Jumps, runs, throws, climbs. Kicks large ball. Squats to play. Puts shoes on part way. Unzips. Fits things together, such as an easy puzzle. Responds rhythmically to music with whole body. • *24 months*: Walks smoothly, watching feet. Runs rhythmically, but unable to start or stop smoothly. Walks up and down stairs alone without alternating feet. Tip toes for a few steps. Pushes tricycle.				
24+	• distinguishes between finger and spoon foods • highly mobile • can walk up stairs without hand being held • can jump from bottom step • can jump in place • can throw a ball • continues to refine movements	• child can use a straw • holds small glass in one hand, replaces glass without dropping • uses spoon correctly but with some spilling • begins to use fork, holds it in fist	• uses sucking pattern and active internal jaw stabilization without biting edge of cup • internal stabilization occurs most of the time during drinking • slight up-down jaw motions or holding edge of cup with teeth may also occur • slight lateral movements	• used on a free, sweeping motion to clean food from upper or lower lips • tongue elevation and depression are independent of jaw movement • skillful tongue tip action may be present • uses tongue tip elevation for swallowing • can transfer food rapidly and skillfully from center to side, from side to	• easy lip closure, with no loss of liquid during drinking or when the cup is removed from the lips • swallows with no loss of saliva or food • swallows solid foods, including those with a combination of textures, with easy lip closure as needed • adequate lip movement during chewing • can keep lips closed

Months	Developmental Motor Milestones	Motoric Development Underlying Feeding	Developmental Milestones of the Jaw	Developmental Milestones of the Tongue	Developmental Milestones of the Lips/Cheeks
24+			of jaw may occur when sucking soft solid or pureed foods from spoon • uses controlled, sustained bite while keeping head at midline when food presented for biting on both sides of mouth • is able to grade opening of jaw when biting foods of various thicknesses • jaw movement in chewing continues to be mixture of nonstereotypic and diagonal rotary movements • circular rotary movements occur when transferring food across midline from one side of mouth to other	center, and from side to side across midline • no extension-retraction movements occur, even with difficult food transfers	during chewing, but does so only when needed to retain the food

Source: Compiled from Alexander, Boehme, and Cupps (1993), Arvedson and Brodsky (1993), Morris and Klein (1987), Owens (1984), Wolf and Glass (1992).

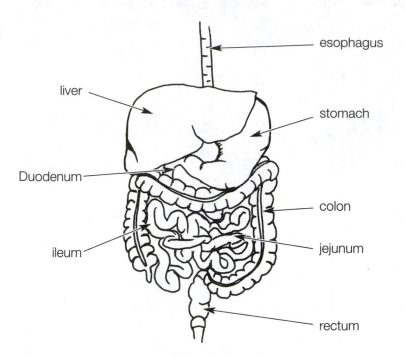

Figure 1–10. Anatomy of the digestive system.

colon where it is eliminated through the rectum (Glass, 1968). Bacteria in the colon react to the nondigestible residue and give the stool its malodorous smell. The newborn infant's stools typically do not smell because of the absence of bacteria in the infant's colon. If they do, this might signal a more serious condition such as bleeding in the GI tract (Batshaw & Perret, 1998).

THE ROLE OF RESPIRATION IN SWALLOWING

Mechanics of Respiration

One of the first lessons that children with dysphagia teach us is that, when given the choice of breathing or feeding, children will choose to breathe. Fundamental to successful feeding is adequate respiration. Breathing takes place when muscle contractions increase the volume of the thorax, thereby creating negative pressure in the lungs. Air is literally sucked into them. When inside and outside air pressure are equalized, inspiration stops, and the thoracic volume decreases, passively coupled with the elastic recoil of the chest wall causing the air to rush back out (expiration). In addition to sharing a common border (the tracheoesophageal wall), the respiratory tract and the GI tract communicate at the pharynx. During the swallow, food passes from the oral cavity through the pharynx to the esophagus. The uppermost structure of the trachea, the larynx, must adequately close and move forward to prevent aspiration. Pharyngeal contractions and changes in air pressure must propel the bolus completely into the esophagus before breathing resumes, possibly sucking any residue of food through the larynx, trachea, and eventually the lungs.

The lungs in a newborn infant are proportionally large in comparison to the size of the thorax (Zemlin, 1988). The skeletal framework for breathing is the spinal column, rib cage, and pelvic girdle. Proper positioning of the pelvis is critical for adequate breath support during speech and feeding (see Figure 1–11). A familiar saying (source unknown) can be revised to reflect the importance of proper positioning for feeding: "Feeding therapy starts at the hips, not at the lips." In addition to the need for proper positioning is adequate lung compliance. The alveoli are lined with moist epithelium and can be likened to "tiny air-filled water bubbles" (Zemlin, 1988, p. 39) that have a tendency to collapse when the surface tension of the lungs is increased. Fortunately, pulmonary surfactant, a detergent-like substance, is produced, which helps the alveoli maintain their patency (Zemlin, 1988).

The infant's airway is protected by its anatomical predisposition to feed and through reflexes to protect the lower airway. Swallowing normally occurs during the expiratory cycle. Expiration is temporarily stopped (swallow apnea), followed by the swallow, and the continuation of the expiration (Preiksaitis, Mayrand, Robins, & Diamant, 1992). If material enters the nasopharynx, larynx, trachea, or lungs, the defense reflexes are triggered to clear the food. Some of the airway defense mechanisms are sneezing, coughing, apnea, bradycardia, and bronchoconstriction (Wolf & Glass, 1992). Unexpectorated food or liquid trapped in the lungs is propelled through the mucociliary clearance or lymphatic clearance. Through phagocytosis (cellular ingestion of particles), the alveoli can clear aspirated material through the lymph system (Curtis & Langmore, 1997).

The coordinated relationship between breathing and swallowing can be seen in their functional control. It is not a coincidence that the "centers" that control both respiration and swallowing are housed within the medulla of the brain stem. It is theorized that interneurons between the respiratory center and swallowing center work together to decode sensory input and activate motor commands necessary for coordinating both (Curtis & Langmore, 1997).

Normal and Abnormal Respiratory Patterns

Newborns have been described as "barrel-chested" because of their relatively large thorax and abdomen. Because of this, the loci of movements during respiration are abdominal. The normal infant respiratory pattern from birth to 5 months is called "belly breathing" (Davis, 1987). Infant vocalizations are limited by this respiratory pattern. However, the loci of movements associated with breathing change as the infant grows. As children gain postural stability, learn to move against gravity, and sit without support, their respiratory movement patterns shift from the primarily abdominal to thoracic. Coupled with the disassociation of the head from the shoulder girdle, these changes are believed to facilitate the onset of speech (Davis, 1987). Similarly, infants' patterns of feedings change as they gain greater postural and respiratory stability. Table 1–9 summarizes normal respiratory patterns from birth to 12 months of age. Children with motor disabilities that affect the development of muscle tone, posture, and movements can cause abnormal respiratory patterns that, in turn, affect feeding (Davis, 1987). For example, children with hypotonia compensate for head-neck-trunk instability by hyperextension. This brings the jaw/tongue forward, elevates and rotates the shoulders, and can lead to abnormal respiratory patterns. These include:

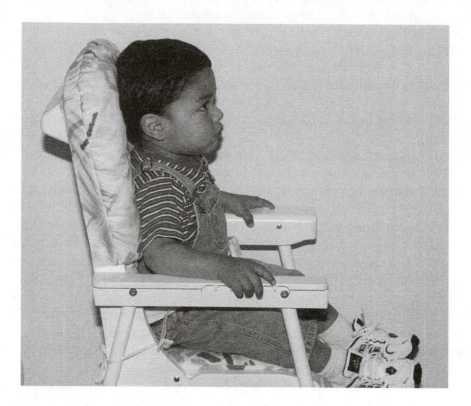

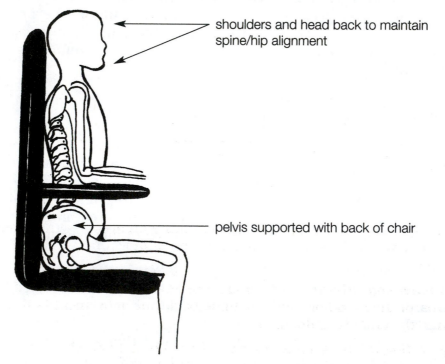

shoulders and head back to maintain spine/hip alignment

pelvis supported with back of chair

Figure 1–11. Proper head, neck, and trunk alignment for feeding. (Adapted from Schuberth [1994].)

TABLE 1–9. Normal Respiratory Patterns from Birth to 12 Months of Age

---

Birth to 5 Months

- belly breathing, 57–80 breaths per minute (BPM)
- greatest movement is in abdomen
- little thoracic movement
- "barrel-chested"
- viscera are compressed/elevated
- cry is short, hypernasal

3–5 Months

- better head control and alignment of head/neck
- stability in larynx allows for longer phonations, cry duration
- primitive weight shift strengthens thoracic musculature
- infant can now resist gravity
- hypernasality reduces after 2 months

6–12 Months

- loci of breathing movements change
- minimal thoracic excursions with greater ribcage expansion
- thorax and viscera move downward
- phonation is longer, greater pitch changes
- loudness control

12 Months and Up

- speech breathing develops
- consistent subglottic air pressure achieved through trunk support
- 41 BPM

Sources: Adapted from Alexander (1987) and Davis (1987).

❖ *belly breathing:* Abdominal expansion during breathing with minimal thoraxic movement. This pattern is considered abnormal in infants 6 months or older.

❖ *gulp breathing:* Short, rapid inhalations that may be associated with extension of the mandible and rhythmic backward movement of the head as though the child is "gulping" air.

❖ *reverse breathing:* A consequence of vertebral instability causing belly breathing, rib cage flaring, and sternal depression.

❖ *irregular/shallow breathing*

❖ *apnea:* Aperiodic cessation of breathing.

During the clinical evaluation of feeding, care must be taken to determine if the feeding disorder is caused by an abnormal respiratory pattern. Muscle tone, rhythm, and patterns of respiration are noted both before and after feedings. Arvedson and Brodsky (1993) recommend the following treatment goals:

❖ establishing head/trunk alignment (see Figures 1–11 and 1–12)

❖ facilitate stability so the child can move against a stable base

❖ provide mobility to improve position and tone for feeding

Effects of Respiration on Sucking/Swallowing

Even in healthy newborn infants, continuous nutritive sucking can slow respiratory rate and affect the infant's oxygenation levels (Shivpuri, Martin, Carlo, & Fanaroff, 1983). There are several ways the newborn respiratory tract can impede airflow through the pharynx, making nipple feeding difficult even for a healthy infant:

❖ Reduced patency of the pharyngeal airway (soft tissues)

❖ Hypopharyngeal compression caused by the position of anatomic structures

❖ Normal physiologic neck flexion

❖ Mandibular excursion (posterior) that reduces the pharyngeal cavity

❖ A small laryngeal vestibule

Breathing through the restricted pharynx, coupled with the cessation of respiration during the normal swallow ("swallow apnea"), is tolerated well by healthy infants. Infants with respiratory compromise, on the other hand, may not tolerate the increased work load of breathing, sucking, and swallowing. Also, during the minute interruptions in breathing while swallowing, they can become bradycardic and hypoxemic. Because nonnutritive sucking on a pacifier (or digit) is not accompanied by regular cessations in the respiratory cycle, it may actually increase oxygenation level in preterm infants (Measel & Anderson, 1979; Paludetto, Robertson, Hack, Shivpuri, & Martin, 1984).

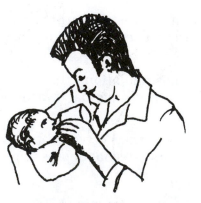

Figure 1–12. Proper feeding position for an infant.

We typically think of infants as "obligate nose breathers" because of their preference for nasal breathing. Because the soft palate rests against the tongue, it was believed that this posture prevented oral breathing in infants (Morris & Klein, 1987). Actually, infants are capable of oral breathing, especially if the nasal passages are occluded (Miller et al., 1985; Rodenstein, Perlmutter, & Stanescu, 1985). Oral breathing, while possible, is not ideal and can lead to consequences in the preterm infant (Wolf & Glass, 1992). More importantly, infants *do not* simultaneously breathe and swallow as reported in earlier literature (cf. Crelin, 1987). At the moment of swallowing, respiration is temporarily suspended. On the other hand, because infants *do* suck and breathe simultaneously, obstruction or compromise of the nasal passages would negatively affect the infant's ability to bottle feed.

Tracheostomy

Some children with upper airway obstruction or other pulmonary complications require a tracheostomy. This surgical procedure involves making an incision or hole in the trachea below the true vocal folds and inserting a tracheostomy tube. The tracheostomy tube has three parts: an outer cannula, inner cannula, and obturator (see Figure 1–13). The outer cannula maintains the opening of the hole, the inner cannula remains in the outer cannula but is removed for cleaning, and the obturator is used to ease initial insertion (Logemann, 1998). Children receiving ventilatory assistance or who are at great aspiration risk typically have cuffed tracheostomy tubes. The cuff is a like a balloon that is inflated to surround the tracheostomy tube and prevent saliva and food from above from penetrating below it into the trachea. When the cuff is deflated, it is similar to a regular tracheostomy tube. If the child can generate enough respiratory power, air from the lungs can pass around the tube and through the larynx for voicing. Children who have difficulty with voicing using a regular tracheostomy tube may need a fenestrated tube. These tubes have a small opening in the top that allows air to pass through into the larynx for voicing (Logemann, 1998).

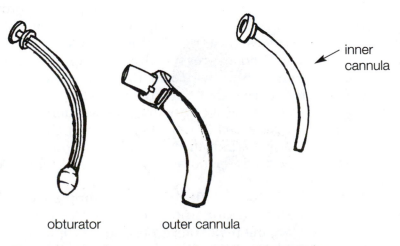

inner
cannula

obturator   outer cannula

Figure 1–13. Components of a tracheostomy tube.

Arvedson and Brodsky (1993) point out that some children receive a tracheostomy as a means of managing their aspiration. Unfortunately, the tracheostomy tube can exacerbate the dysphagia by limiting laryngeal elevation. Furthermore, the cuff may create pressure in the esophagus that disrupts the swallow. Children who have long-term tracheostomy tubes experience reduced airflow through the larynx, with reduced vocal fold closure for swallowing and voicing (Logemann, 1998).

Aspiration Management

Infants and children who are unable to take nutrition orally will receive primary enteral feedings or tube feedings (see Alternate Methods of Nutritional Intake on p. 39). Enteral support can be temporary or long-term, but the tube placement is reversible. There are, however, several permanent surgical procedures designed to manage chronic, uncontrollable aspiration. These are "last ditch efforts" used only if the child is at significant risk of death because of aspiration. Logemann (1998) describes some of these techniques:

1. *epiglottic pull-down:* The epiglottis is sutured to the arytenoid cartilages.

2. *laryngeal bypass or tracheoesophageal diversion:* The trachea and esophagus are separated at about the third tracheal ring. The proximal end is sutured to the cervical esophagus, and the distal end is brought out through a hole in the skin.

3. *total laryngectomy:* The entire larynx and hyoid bone are removed. The trachea is sutured to the base of neck to form a stoma, and the esophagus is sutured to the pharynx. There is complete separation of the trachea and esophagus. This procedure is only done in children who have long-term tracheotomy tubes and who have severe laryngeal dysfunction without possibility of ever attaining laryngeal voicing.

PHYSIOLOGY OF THE SUCK-SWALLOW-BREATHE SEQUENCE

Physiology of Sucking

For infants to attain liquid from a nipple, they must adequately compress the nipple between the tongue and the hard palate to squeeze liquid out. Logan and Bosma (1967) speculated that the ridges running horizontally along the hard palate help keep the nipple in position. Fluid expression from a nipple is also accomplished through the creation of negative pressure in the oral cavity. Here, the lip seal around the nipple completely closes the oral cavity. When the tongue and mandible drop, this increases the size of the oral cavity and, subsequently, creates a pressure differential between the positive pressure in the bottle and the negative pressure in the oral cavity. The liquid is "sucked" from the nipple into the mouth. Both compression and changes in pressure are responsible for successful nipple feeding (Logan & Bosma, 1967; Matthew, 1991).

According to Morris and Klein (1987), the infant's nipple feeding progresses developmentally from suckling to sucking and is characterized by changes in tongue movement patterns and degree of lip closure around the nipple. In each, nipple compression and pressure changes draw liquid from the nipple. The way this is achieved, however, changes as the infant develops. By about 6 months of age, the infant's facial growth and transition from physiologic flexion to more stable head/neck/trunk support has allowed an increase in the intraoral space and tongue mobility. The suckling seen in young infants, which is a product of restricted intraoral space, reduced tongue movements, and sensorimotor development, gradually develops into a more mature sucking pattern by about 9 months of age (see Figure 1–14). It should be noted that the distinction between sucking and suckling patterns varies in the literature (cf. Morris & Klien, 1987; Wolf & Glass, 1992), and not all authors differentiate these terms. In this text, the term "suck(l)ing" will be used when referring to either sucking or suckling. Otherwise, the terms "suckling" and "sucking" will be used and specifically refer to:

Suckling

❖ birth–6 months
❖ loose lips, reduced lip seal, tongue seals around the nipple
❖ wide mandibular excursions
❖ tongue moves in/out

Sucking

❖ 6–9 months onward
❖ tight lip seal, reduced tongue seal
❖ reduced mandibular excursions
❖ tongue moves up/down

Nutritive and Nonnutritive Suck(l)ing

Suck(l)ing for nutrition (nutritive suck/suckle [NS]) or suck(l)ing on a pacifier or nipple that does not deliver nutrition (nonnutritive suck/suckle [NNS]) are both very important for infant development. The purpose of NS is to obtain nutrition. It not only provides the early oral motor experiences that are essential for oral sensorimo-

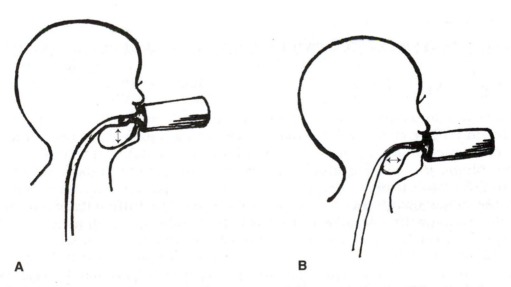

A   **B**

Figure 1–14. Drawing of suckling versus sucking movements of the tongue. **A.** During sucking, the tongue moves in an up-down direction, with opening/closing movements of the jaw. **B.** During suckling, the tongue moves in an in-out direction, with more open/closing of the jaw. (Adapted from Arvedson and Brodsky [1993].)

tor development but also is an opportunity for the early establishment of child/caregiver bonding (Bosma, 1990). On the other hand, NNS in healthy newborns is calming, state regulating, and pacifies (hence the name "pacifier") the child's need to suck(le). Nonnutritive suck(l)ing in medically fragile children, especially those who are receiving primary enteral feedings, helps them to adapt to new environments, self-stabilize, increase oxygen saturation levels, and increase feeding performance (McCain, 1995; Pickler, Frankel, Walsch, & Thompson, 1996). In addition, children who are allowed to nonnutritively suck(le) while receiving tube feedings have faster gastric emptying, gain weight faster, are better at regulating state, and ultimately leave the NICU sooner (Bernbaum, Pereria, Watkins, & Perckham, 1983; Field et al., 1982; Measel & Anderson, 1979).

NNS is typically twice as fast as the NS (NNS = 2 per second vs. NS = 1 per second). This difference is probably caused by the interjection and coordination of respiration after each NS, which slows nutritive sucking rate. Wolfe (1968) reported the rate of suck(l)ing per second of NNS and NS rates in preterm infants (37–38 weeks) to 9-month-old infants. NNS rates increased from 1.7 to 2.7. NS rates increased from .92 to 1.5. In the healthy infant, NS and NNS occur in rhythmic, organized patterns called "bursts." In the NNS burst, the infant suck(le)s 6–8 times before pausing to swallow. Breathing is continuous and regular throughout the NNS and only interrupted by the swallow. With age, the NNS burst increases. In NS, there are typically 20–30 cycles of suck(le)-swallow-breathe, followed by a pause of about 5 seconds for "catch-up breaths." The burst pattern and the ratio of suck(le)-swallow-breathe are influenced by the type of nipple and flow rate (Matthew, 1991). However, most infants begin with a suck(le)-swallow-breathe ratio of 1:1:1. As the feeding comes to an end, this ratio may increase to 2:1:1. The most important issue is not the ratio (i.e., 2 or 1 suck[le]s per swallow), rather, it is whether the infant can establish *and maintain* a rhythmic suck(l)ing pattern.

Immature Suckling Patterns

NNS in the preterm infant 27–28 weeks postconceptional age (PCA) is very disorganized and arrhythmic, characterized by single suckles followed by long and variable pauses (Hack, Estabrook, & Robertson, 1985; Palmer & Heyman, 1993). Immature suckling patterns of 3–5 suckles per burst, followed by a respiratory pause and swallows before and after suckles, have been documented at 32 3/7 weeks PCA (Weber, Woolridge, & Baum, 1986). Suckles are typically slow (1.5 per second), and pauses continue to be variable. As the preterm infant or full-term medically fragile infant matures, the occurrence and duration of suckling bursts-pause cycles increase and become "transitional" (Palmer, 1993). Transitional suckling patterns are also disorganized and characterized by 5–10 suckles per burst. These longer bursts may be accompanied by periods of feeding-induced apnea, which further complicate the feeding (Palmer, 1993).

One instrument that can be used to assess suckling patterns is the Neonatal Oral-Motor Assessment Scale or NOMAS® (Palmer, 1993). The NOMAS examines jaw and tongue movements during feeding into three categories: normal, disorganized, and dysfunctional. The NOMAS®, presented in Section 3, can be used as a resource when evaluating suckling patterns in infants. To reliably use this scale, however, certification is required (Palmer, April 1999, personal communication).

Readiness To Feed

The ability to sustain oral nutrition is usually one of the necessary criteria for discharge from the hospital to home (Gale, 2000). There is no one sign to indicate when a preterm or medically fragile infant is ready to start NS. There is, however, one general rule:

> If an infant can produce a NNS, she or he *may* or *may not* demonstrate a normal NS. Conversely, if an infant does not demonstrate a normal NNS, she or he *will not* exhibit a normal NS and is not yet ready for oral feedings.

Oral feedings are not recommended in premature infants until they weigh at least 1500 grams, are without significant pulmonary problems, and are 34 weeks (Bu'Lock, Woolridge, & Baum, 1990; Kinner & Beachy, 1994) or at the very earliest 33 weeks PCA (Roberston & Bhatia, 1993). Although it is true that infants in utero begin NNS sucking and swallowing amniotic fluid during the second trimester as early as 12–14 weeks PCA (Bosma, 1985), their ability to coordinate suck-swallow-breathe is not fully developed before 33 weeks PCA (Roberston & Bhatia, 1993). Even if infants can make some attempt to orally feed before this time, the result of their disorganized feeding attempts is often a great expenditure of energy, and subsequently, their "feeding" is counterproductive to gaining weight (McCain, 1995). Other research supports this assertion and suggests that 31- to 33-week-old infants who are "successfully" orally fed small amounts of liquid via nipple (5 ml) are not necessarily successful with larger volumes (Gale, 2000). Furthermore, continual attempts to nipple feed medically fragile infants who are not ready to feed orally may actually extend the length of their hospital stay (Gale, 2000).

Nipple readiness signs are (Gale, 2000):

❖ physiologic stability

❖ alertness levels

❖ successful NNS

McCain (1995) also suggests that monitoring behavioral state before and during feeding may be a better way to predict feeding readiness and success rather than infant heart rate.

BRAIN STEM AND CORTICAL CONTROL OF DEGLUTITION

Eliciting the Swallowing Response

Early literature refers to swallowing as a reflex because it was thought to be a chain of simple peripheral reflexes triggered by a series of sensory inputs as the bolus moved from the oral cavity into the pharynx (Bosma, 1967; Logemann, 1998). Although swallowing can be reflexively evoked (involuntary swallowing), this is not a part of voluntary deglutition (Miller, 1986). One example of an involuntary swallow is seen in the Santmyer swallow reflex. This reflexive swallow is elicited by a puff of air onto the infant's face and is used to aid the insertion of nasogastric tubes, "force" a swallowing during behavioral feeding therapy, and help during videofluoroscopic evaluations of swallowing (Walter, 1994). It is present in preterm infants (33–34 weeks) and typically disappears by 2 years of age (Omari et al. 1995; Orenstein, Giarrusso, Proujansky, & Kocosis, 1988).

The process of voluntary swallowing for nutrition, on the other hand, is much more complex than could be executed by a string of simple reflexes. The act of swallowing is now believed to be a cortical and brain stem mediated response, or central program, that once activated, sends motor commands to the muscles of deglutition in a highly coordinated sequence (Perlman & Christersen, 1997). Swallowing requires:

❖ a large area of brain stem

❖ six cranial nerves

❖ a large number of sensory receptors

❖ thirty-one pairs of muscles

The normal "swallowing response" is initiated or "triggered" by sensory input coming from the oral and pharyngeal cavities. Figure 1–15 shows the sensory and motor controls of swallowing. Table 1–10 summarizes the neural control of swallowing.

To trigger a swallow, sensory information must be sent and "decoded" by the swallowing center within the brain stem. In infants, the input is in the form of touch, liquids, or soft pressure to the soft palate, anterior faucial pillars, dorsum of tongue, and valleculae (Bosma, 1985). Taste alone is not sufficient to elicit swallow-

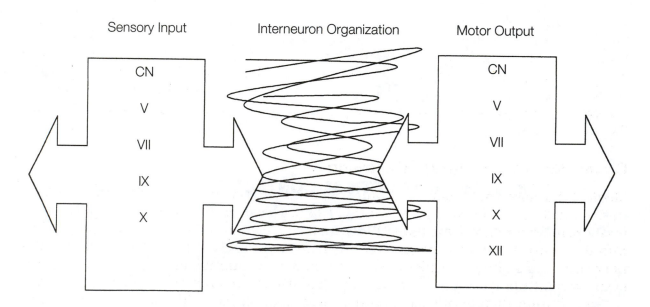

Figure 1–15. Schematic representation of the swallowing center. When the appropriate sensory input comes into the swallowing center from cranial nerves V, VII, IX, and X, the swallow response is "triggered" and carried out by motor commands (motor output) to the muscles of deglutition from cranial nerves V, VII, IX, X, and XII.

TABLE 1–10. Functional Control of Swallowing in Infants

- Swallowing is a property of a precisely interconnected set of neurons. It depends on the activity of the brain stem neurons that belong to a functionally defined "swallowing center."

- The swallowing center is located in the brain stem and two primary sites in the prefrontal cortex. The bulk of the work of swallowing takes place in the brain stem

  → The NTS is the sensory recognition center in the medulla. It decodes the message and sends it to the nucleus ambiguus (in the reticular formation) via interneurons that then initiate a pharyngeal swallow.

  → The two regions of the NTS and NA that are responsible for swallowing are located bilaterally in the brain stem and are heavily interconnected. This ensures accuracy of bilateral motor activity and proper sequencing of muscles involved in swallowing.

  → The neurons that program the swallow response for the pharyngeal/esophageal stages are in the brain stem. However, bilateral cortical areas are important for evoking the initiation of swallowing.

  → The brain stem contains the interneurons necessary for carrying out a successful swallow. The cortex has input that is helpful, but not essential, for the initiation of the response.

ing. Although it is true that infants can detect varying degrees of sweetness and may show a preference (or aversion) to a brand of formula, switching formulas will not improve swallowing function in infants with motor-based swallowing problems.

In young to middle-aged adults, the swallowing response is triggered at the anterior faucial pillars (Logemann, 1998). Because of the high position of the valleculae in the neck of the infant, swallowing is typically triggered at the level of the valleculae. Beecher (1994) notes that infants progress from a tongue back-down motion to elicit a swallow response to a tongue back-up motion. In the tongue back-down motion, the base of the tongue moves backward, dropping the bolus into the pharynx where the response is triggered at the level of the valleculae. As the child ages, the neck elongates and the larynx descends. The response now is triggered by the tongue moving backward and upward to press against the anterior faucial pillars (Beecher, 1994).

Cranial Nerves in Feeding/Swallowing

Medical diseases that isolate and affect specific cranial nerves in children resulting in dysphagia are relatively rare (Walter, 1994). However, the presence or absence of many primitive reflexes mediated by cranial nerves can indicate the integrity of the infant's central nervous system (CNS). Lefton-Greif (1997) suggests that cranial nerve screening should be included in the clinical evaluation of pediatric feeding and swallowing. Ruling out CNS damage, particularly cranial nerve (CN) damage, is critical to accurate therapeutic intervention. For example, a child who is not establishing a rhythmic sucking pattern because of fatigue will be treated very differently from a child with Vernet's syndrome, where tongue weakness is caused by damage to CN XII. Neurologically based feeding disorders are presented in Section 2, and procedures for evaluating cranial nerve function are presented in Section 3.

DEVELOPMENTAL FEEDING SKILLS

Normal Feeding Development

Feeding specialists who are treating children with dysphagia must make decisions regarding when to introduce new textures and utensils. Each child must be evaluated individually; however, there is a general progression of normal feeding. In fact, there is evidence to suggest that children have "sensitive periods" for feeding development in which they are best ready to learn or adapt to new stimuli, in this case food textures and utensils (Illingworth & Lister, 1964). For example, failing to transition from bottle to spoon feeding around 6 months of age can lead to long-term aversion of solids or textures (Illingworth & Lister, 1964; Stevenson & Allaire, 1991). Meer (1998) suggests that normally developing bottle-fed infants should begin receiving puree consistencies from a spoon no later than 4 months of age (breast fed is 6 months of age). Conversely, puree consistencies should *not* be presented before 4 months of age because of the risk of developing food allergies or, in rare cases, methemoglobinemia, a condition that can lead to death. Ironically, some caregivers of healthy infants attempt to thicken bottle feedings by adding puree consistencies or more commonly rice cereal. The belief is that thickening formula improves the caloric intake, increases sleeping time, and decreases crying time, thereby allowing the infant to gain, rather than lose, weight (Tuchman & Walter, 1994).

Historically, thickening feedings has been considered a conventional approach to treat gastroesophageal reflux (Tuchman & Walter, 1994; Wolf & Glass, 1992). The rationale is that the heavy, bulkier food would remain in the stomach rather than reflux back into the esophagus. However, research suggests that thickening bottle fed formula or breast milk with puree consistencies, especially cereals, does *not* improve infants' sleeping patterns or help establish normal feeding behaviors (Meer, 1998). Although thickening food may be effective in reducing episodes of emesis, it does not appear to reduce episodes of reflux (Orenstein, Magill, & Brooks, 1987).

Whereas Table 1–8 follows feeding development as it co-develops with motor development, Appendix B (see p. 215) presents feeding as it co-develops with cognition, sensory integration, socialization, and communication.

Nutritional Needs of Infants and Children

Most newborn infants need between 2.5–4.5 ounces of formula every 3–4 hours or breast milk every 2–3 hours. By 4 months of age, infants take in about 6–8 ounces per feeding. Expected caloric intakes are presented in Table 1–11. When treating children with dysphagia, the primary goal is to facilitate proper nutrition and hydration. Often, children with long-term feeding problems need additional help maintaining or gaining weight. Table 1–12 provides suggestions for increasing calories to children's diets.

Parents/caregivers of children with dysphagia monitor oral intake not only by calories but also volume such as cubic centimeter (cc), teaspoon (tsp), tablespoon (tbsp), and ounce (oz). The following are important conversions you will want to remember:

1 cc	1 ml
1 tsp	5 ml
1 tbsp	15 ml
1 oz	30 ml

TABLE 1–11. General Feeding Progression

Age (in Months)	Presentation	Recommended Food Type	Oral Motor Skills	Ways To Help the Child Transition
Birth–4	Nipple	Breast milk or formula	Suckling becomes sucking	1. Position the infant so that the hips are flexed, chin is tucked down (but not to chest). 2. Move the shoulders forward with the arm toward the face/bottle
4–6	Nipple, spoon	Breast milk or formula, iron-fortified cereal mixed with breast milk or formula	Mature sucking pattern, sucking from spoon	1. Present the spoon tip horizontally to the tongue; avoid scraping of gum/teeth. 2. Encourage lip closure and food removal by applying light pressure.
6–8	Nipple, spoon, cup introduced (8 months)	Breast milk or formula; commercial pureed baby foods or pureed table foods (no sugar or salt added); new grains introduced	Primitive reflexes are diminishing (rooting, biting); munching/chewing solids	1. Allow infant to bite or suck liquid from the cup with the tongue. 2. Encourage chin down; do not allow the head to go back when introducing the cup. 3. Hold the cup to corners of the mouth; avoid "dumping" liquid into the mouth.
8–12	Nipple, spoon, cup; self-feeding without utensils	Breast milk, formula, nonacidic juices (apple, pear, grape), finger foods (crackers, bread, pasta, cereal), meat and other finely chopped proteins introduced (ground meat, cheese, legumes, egg yolks)	Upper lip used to clean spoon, tongue lateralization begins, biting on objects	1. Seat the child in a high chair with head, neck, and spine aligned, hips back against chair, feet supported, arms free.
12–15	Nipple (weaning), cup, spoon, self-feeding without utensil	Liquids, pureed, chopped fine solids, coursely chopped table foods (15 months)	Tongue lateralization, rotary chew emerges	1. Seat the child in a high chair with head, neck, and spine aligned, hips back against chair, feet supported, arms free.
15–24	Cup, self-feeding with utensils (fork/spoon)	Table foods	Rotary chew, increased jaw stability in cup drinking	1. Start by allowing the child to guide the feeder's hand with spoon to the mouth to taking control of spoon. 2. Help the child to hold the spoon handle with a straight wrist to control food in spoon bowl.

Sources: Compiled from Arveson and Brodsky (1993), Morris and Klein (1987).

TABLE 1–12. How To Add Calories to a Child's Diet

1. Use commercial infant formulas for premature infants. These generally carry 24 calories/ounce instead of the standard 20.

2. Increase the caloric density of infant formulas by:
   - reducing the amount of water added to concentrated or powdered formulas
   - adding glucose or fat to ready-to-feed infant formulas (fat should not exceed more than 50% of calories)

   Important: If left to stand for a long period of time, fat in the formula will separate. This is of concern for a child who may be aspirating.

   Important: Final caloric density of the formula should not exceed 30 calories/ounce.

   Important: The presence of sugar or fat in the stool, high urine-specific gravity, vomiting, and/or diarrhea are all indications of poor tolerance to the high calorie load.

3. *Butter and margarine:* (45 calories/1 tsp) use extra on crackers, toast, vegetables, cooked cereals, and soups.

4. *Granola:* (125 calories/ ¼ cup) use in cookies, muffins, and bread batters. Sprinkle on vegetables, yogurt, ice cream, pudding, custard, and fruit. Mix with dry fruits and nuts for snacks.

5. *Honey:* (65 calories/1 tbsp) use as a glaze for meals or add to breads, cereals, beverages, and desserts.

6. *Infant rice cereal:* (15 calories/1 dry tbsp) add to casseroles, meat loaf, cream soups, and mashed potatoes.

7. *Jelly or jam:* (50 calories/1 tbsp) use plenty on breads, hot cereals, or as an ingredient in a milk drink.

8. *Nonfat dried milk solids:* (15 calories/1 dry tbsp) add to mashed potatoes, whole milk, and other milk drinks as well as to casseroles, meat loaf, and cream soups.

9. *Potato flakes:* (13 calories/1 dry tbsp) see infant rice cereal for uses.

10. *Powdered nondairy creamer:* (11 calories/1 tbsp) use in gravies, soups, milkshakes, and hot cereals.

11. *Sour cream:* (30 calories/1 tbsp) use on vegetables, in gravies, or as a salad dressing.

12. *Sugar, brown:* (50 calories/1 tbsp) add to hot cereal, sprinkle on toast, or use as a coating on fresh fruit pieces.

13. *Sugar, granulated:* (45 calories/1 tbsp) similar uses to brown sugar.

14. *Vegetable oil:* (45 calories/1 tbsp) use to sauté or fry foods. Add to milk drinks.

15. *Wheat germ, toasted:* (27 calories/1 tbsp) add to casseroles, cereal, and bread-type products.

16. *Whipping topping sweetened:* (10 calories/1 tbsp) use on hot beverages, desserts, and fruits.

17. *Whipping cream, heavy:* (52 calories/1 tbsp) add to fruit, puddings, hot chocolate, gelatin dessert, and other desserts.

High Calorie Beginning Table Foods

yogurt	tuna or meat salad
pudding	liverwurst
cottage cheese	scrambled egg
pancakes	cheese
french fries	mashed avocado
hot cereal made with milk, margarine added	

Suggestions Regarding Feeding

- Include at least one food the child likes at each meal.
- Consider the texture and preferences your child has.
- Offer high calorie snacks but limit those that are high in fat because they can cause a decrease in appetite.
- Serve food at regular times each day.
- Offer young children 4–6 meals/snacks per day every 2–4 hours.

Do not allow the child to nibble food or drink beverages throughout the day. This may decrease the child's appetite or not allow him/her to feel "hungry."

Source: Compiled from Richard (1991).

ALTERNATE METHODS OF NUTRITIONAL INTAKE

Primary and Supplemental Enteral Support

"Enteral support" or "gavage feeding" refers to tube feeding. Ultimately it is the family, on the physician's advice, who makes the decision regarding the placement and type of tube feeding the child will receive. The following is a summary of the different types of tube feedings, advantages, and disadvantages.

Orogastric Tubes	❖ Inserted via mouth through the pharynx, esophagus, and into the stomach.
Advantages	❖ Used in premature infants and eliminates the risk for potential obstruction of the nasal airway.
	❖ Provides short-term nutritional maintenance.
Disadvantages	❖ Interference with lip closure and tongue function
	❖ Presence of a foreign body in the pharynx and esophagus.
Nasogastric Tubes	❖ Inserted into one side of the nose into the pharynx and through the esophagus into the stomach.
	❖ Typically, a new tube is replaced every 3–4 days.
Advantages	❖ Provides short-term nutritional maintenance.
	❖ May be replaced with a gastrostomy tube if supplemental nutritional needs prove to be long term.
Disadvantages	❖ Inability to completely close off the soft palate may result in reduced intraoral pressure needed for effective sucking and swallowing.
Nasoduodenal Tubes	❖ Inserted into the nasal cavity, through the pharynx, guided into the esophagus and through the stomach into the duodenum.
	❖ Used when reflux is a problem.
	❖ Used for long-term feeding problems
Nasojejunal Tubes	❖ Inserted into the nasal cavity, through the pharynx, guided into the esophagus and through the stomach into the jejunum.
Advantages	❖ Used for long-term feeding problems
Disadvantages	❖ Inability to completely close off the soft palate may result in reduced intraoral pressure needed for effective sucking and swallowing.

There may be a reduction in the protective gag function because of sensory adaptation when a tube is left in place for a long period of time. Other complications may include emesis, gastroesophageal reflux, delayed gastric emptying, and nasal/pharyngeal irritation. Finally, there is a strong possibility that the negative stimulation associated with inserting and removing nasally inserted tubes cause a situation for development of oral aversion, with significant implications relating to the development of oral-motor feeding skills.

Gastrostomy Tubes	❖ G-tubes or percutaneous endoscopic gastrostomy (PEG) tubes
	❖ Inserted into the stomach

Advantages	❖ The area of invasion is away from the mouth and may permit the infant to discover pleasant oral sensation faster.
	❖ Provides nutritional support for long-term feeding problems.
Disadvantages	❖ Often causes reflux and may require further surgery to reduce gastroesophageal reflux (see Table 1–13).
	❖ There can be leakage around the tube site.
Jejunostomy Tubes	❖ J-tubes or percutaneous jejunostomy tubes (PEJ)
	❖ Inserted into the jejunum (the portion of the small intestine between the duodenum and ileum)
Advantages	❖ Area of insertion is away from the mouth and may permit the infant to discover pleasant oral sensation faster.
	❖ Less likely to cause reflux
Disadvantages	❖ Requires specially formulated liquid nutrition
	❖ There can be leakage around the tube site.
Gastrostomy-Jejunostomy Tube	❖ G-J tube
	❖ A connected tube with one end inserted into the stomach and the other into the jejunum.
Advantages	❖ Allows for removal of stomach contents and nutrition delivered to the jejunum.
Disadvantages	❖ More invasive procedure
	❖ Increases the chances of leakage around tube sites.

TABLE 1–13. Surgical Management of Reflux in Children

Belsy Mark IV: The esophageal hiatus is narrowed by two rows of sutures between the fundus of the stomach and the esophagus. The upper part of the stomach is wrapped 270° around the anterior portion of the esophagus (a.k.a. plication of the stomach around the esophagus).

Nissen fundoplication: This procedure is similar to the Belsy Mark IV with the exception that the upper part of the stomach is wrapped a full 360° around the esophagus. This results in a slightly higher pressure against the upper esophageal segment than the Belsy Mark IV. A laparoscopic Nissen procedure, sometimes referred to as the "floppy" Nissen fundoplication, is becoming more popular. With either approach, there is a greater risk of postoperative dypshagia due to difficulty belching or vomiting if the repair is too tight.

Hill posterior gastropexy and calibration of the cardia: Fixation or "anchoring" of the posterior portion of the stomach with adjustment or "calibration" of the lower esophageal sphinctor. The gastroesophgeal junctions are sutured to create a partial wrap around the enterance of the esophagus into the stomach.

Collis gastroplasty: Chronic reflux can result in esophageal strictures that must be surgically removed, thereby shortening the esophagus. In the Collis gastroplasty, the esophagus is "lengthened" by cutting a tube of stomach as a continuation of the esophagus. This procedure is typically followed by a full fundoplication.

Thal fundic patch operation: A surgical procedure to repair reflux-induced esophageal strictures. A longitudinal cut is made across the stricture allowing it to spread open. A skin graft is applied across the opening. This procedure is followed by a full fundoplication.

Sources: Kamolz, T., Bammer, T., and Pointer, R. (2000). Predictability of dysphagia after laparoscopic Nissen fundoplication. *The American Journal of Gastroenterology, 95,* 408–414. Sabiston, D. (1986). *Textbook of surgery* (12th ed., p. 765). Philadelphia, PA: W.B. Saunders Company. Ogorek, C. (1995). Gastroesophageal reflux disease. In J. Berk (Ed.), *Bockus gastroenterology* (pp. 445–463). Philadelphia, PA: W.B. Saunders Company.

OVERVIEW OF THE NEONATAL INTENSIVE CARE UNIT

Neonatal Intensive Care Nursery Levels

The Intensive Care Nursery (ICN) can be categorized into three levels. Most hospitals have a Level 1 ICN treating minor problems in generally "healthy" infants. Discharge is typically 1–5 days. Level 1 has the highest staff/patient ratios.

A Level 2 ICN treats low birth weight (LBW) premature or full-term infants. Traditionally, LBW is defined as less than 2500 grams but some hospitals consider LBW to be infants weighing less than 1500 grams. Level 2 ICNs are also called "step-down" or "feeder-grower" units. Discharge is typically 1 to several months. Level 3 ICNs provide the highest intervention with surgical cases, very low birth weight infants (VLBW <1000 grams), and extremely low birth weight (ELBW < 800 grams) medically fragile premature infants. Level 3 has the lowest staff/patient ratios and the most equipment, such as high-pressure and oscillating vents and extracorporeal membrane oxygenation (ECMO). ECMO is a highly invasive procedure used for full-term infants with severe respiratory problems. It removes carbon dioxide and provides oxygen to the blood by directly passing the infant's blood through a heart-lung bypass machine.

Interdisciplinary Team

When working with infants and older children with dysphagia, a number of different professionals collaborate to provide an individualized treatment plan. SLPs could work with the following:

Family: Pediatric dysphagia therapy is a family-centered therapy. It focuses on the needs of the child within her or his most immediate social unit—the family.

Neonatologist: A pediatrician with advanced knowledge of intensive care newborn medicine. A Fellow is a pediatrician training to become a neonatologist. A Resident is a physician in training.

Pediatrician: A physician specializing in pediatric medicine.

Gastroenterologist: A physician specializing in diagnosing and treating disorders of the digestive tract.

OTR/RPT: Registered occupational and physical therapists.

Nutritionist: Monitors the child's nutritional needs.

Nurse: Primary nurse or neonatal nurse practitioner.

Radiologist: A physician who will be involved in all diagnostic imaging (CT, VFSS, upper GI, etc.)

Social Worker: Newborn Unit Social Worker. An individual with a masters degree in social work who is involved in the multidisciplinary team management of patients and their families. The social worker is responsible for patient advocacy, ensuring high-quality patient care, assessment treatment planning, and patient/family education. In some hospitals, the social worker also can be involved in discharge planning.

ENT: An otolaryngologist, a physician who specializes in diseases of the ear, nose, and throat

Psychologist: A professional whose primary focus is on the assessment and treatment of human behavior.

Surgeon: A physician specializing in the surgical treatment of diseases, injuries, or deformities.

Pulmonologist: A physician specializing in diseases of the lungs.

Dentist: A person with a Doctorate in Dental Surgery who specializes in the care of the teeth and surrounding tissues and the correction of malocclusion.

Respiratory Therapist: A professional who specializes in the practice of respiratory care.

Lactation Consultant: A professional who specializes in breast feeding, pumping, and storing breast milk.

Neonatal Individualized Developmental Care and Assessment Program

The Neonatal Individualized Developmental Care and Assessment Program (NIDCAP) is a program designed to maximize the developmental outcomes of preterm infants. NIDCAP is founded in the Synactive Theory of Neurobehavioral Development (Als, 1982). This theory describes four developmental subsystems: (a) autonomic, (b) motor, (c) state control, (d) interactive and self-regulation. The subsystems emerge interdependently during the fetal period of gestation. Self-regulation refers to the infant's ability to maintain neurodevelopmetal balance within the environment. The NIDCAP modifies the NICU to provide a climate conducive to neurobehavioral development. NICU personnel must go through extensive training (approximately 1 year) to become NIDCAP certified. Reducing exposure to light and noise, minimizing handling so that the infant can rest, improving infant positioning to increase flow of blood to the brain, and educating the parents and family on how to recognize and minimize infant stressors are some of the modifications that NIDCAP enforces. The benefits of NIDCAP include (a) decreased occurrence of intraventricular hemorrhaging, (b) shorter duration of ventilator support, (c) shorter duration of hospitalization, and (d) improved ability to nipple feed in fewer days (Brown & Heermann, 1997; Tribotti & Stein, 1992).

Monitoring Physiologic Function

Neonatal Technology

The development of computerized systems resulted in the commercialization of intensive care monitoring equipment and networks for the hospital NICU. Presently, NICUs make use of an extensive number of medical instruments to monitor and treat premature infants. A typical NICU bed consist of the following instruments (see Figure 1–16):

Life Support

- ❖ Incubator
- ❖ Ventilator
- ❖ Extracorporeal membraneous oxygenation (ECMO) system
- ❖ Infusion pumps

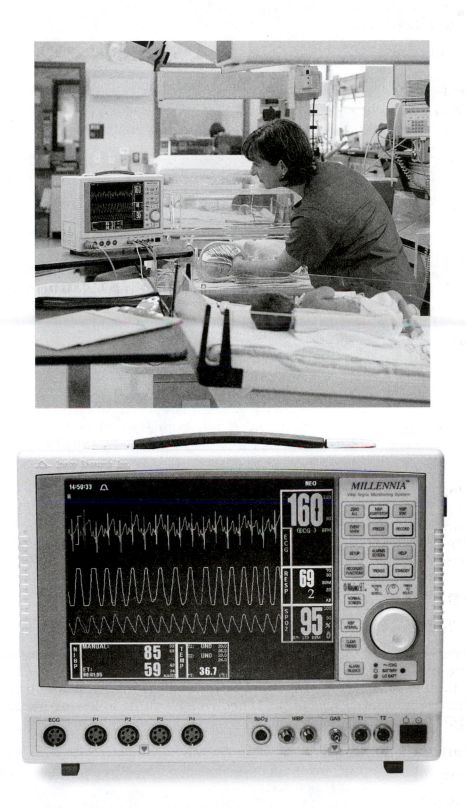

Figure 1–16. Equipment commonly used in the NICU.

Monitoring

❖ Temperature monitor

❖ ECG monitor

❖ Blood oxygen saturation monitor

❖ Pressure monitors

❖ Apnea monitors

Equipment in the NICU

The following is a listing of some of the equipment in the NICU and a description of what it is used for:

Apnea and bradycardia monitor: If the baby's breathing and heart rate become abnormal, an alarm will sound, alerting the NICU staff. These machines only record the baby's heart and breathing rates; they do not control them. Apnea is cessation of breathing that lasts longer than 20 seconds. Bradycardia is when the heart rate drops below 80 beats per minute.

Bililights: A row of fluorescent lights that are placed over the baby's incubator or warmer. Also called "Phototherapy," it helps infants with hyperbillirubinemia (jaundice); bililights break down the bilirubin so that the infant can excrete the bilirubin found beneath the skin. The infant wears protective patches over the eyes.

Blood pressure monitor: Blood pressure may be measured periodically by a small cuff placed around the infant's arm or leg or continuously by a catheter placed in an artery.

Cardiac monitor: A noninvasive machine that provides a recording of the electrical conduction of the heart by electrodes placed on the infants chest, abdomen, arms, or legs. An alarm system is activated if the heart rate rises above (tachycardia) or falls below (bradycardia) preset levels. Many cardiac monitors also display respiratory rate, blood pressure, and oxygen saturation levels. Be aware that the readings from most monitors are delayed and represent an average over 6–10 seconds from the actual timed event (see Figure 1–16).

Continuous positive airway pressure (CPAP): The administration of oxygen and air under pressure through short two-pronged tubes placed in the nose. It improves oxygenation by opening alveoli and promoting the effective exchange of oxygen and carbon dioxide.

Endotracheal tube: A thin plastic tube inserted through the infant's mouth or nose into the trachea to allow delivery of air/oxygen to the lungs via a respirator. It is secured with tape and attaches by tubing to a respirator.

Extracorporeal membrane oxygenation (ECMO): A highly invasive procedure that removes carbon dioxide and provides oxygen to the blood by directly passing the infant's blood through a heart-lung bypass machine.

Feeding pump: A machine that delivers a preset amount of enteral feeding to an infant at a preset rate through a gavage or gastrostomy tube. An alarm system is activated if obstruction of flow of the enteral feeding is detected.

Heart monitor: When the infant's heart rate slows down, messages travel through the electrodes and will set of an alarm which alerts the NICU staff.

Incubator: A heated plastic box. It will help keep the infant warm and isolated from germs within the NICU.

IV (intravenous infusion): This is a needle, or small tube, that is placed into one of the veins of the infant. It is attached by tubing to a container of fluid.

IV pump: A machine that delivers a preset amount of IV fluids, medications, or nutrition at a preset rate into a vein. An alarm system is activated if obstruction of flow of fluid is detected.

Nasal prongs: Small tubes placed inside the infant's nostrils to provide a steady stream of oxygen. If the oxygen is delivered under pressure, it is known as **continuous positive airway pressure (CPAP).**

Oxygen hood: A clear plastic box placed over the infant's head. Oxygen flows into it via a tube attached to a source of oxygen. Generally used for infants who are breathing on their own but still need extra oxygen.

Oxygen mask: A mask placed over the infant's mouth and nose. Oxygen flows through a tube and into the mask at a constant rate.

Positive end expiration pressure (PEEP): A machine to maintain a constant pressure to the alveoli, keep alveoli open at all times, and promote effective oxygen and carbon dioxide exchange. Similar to CPAP (see above), but involves more direct access to the lungs, thus providing better gas exchange.

Pulse oximeter: The "pulse ox" is a noninvasive machine that measures the amount of saturated oxygen in the infant's blood by a sensor clipped to a palm, foot, toe, or wrist. An alarm system is activated if oxygen saturation falls below a preset level.

Respirator: A machine used to provide partial or full respiratory support. Also known as a ventilator.

Suction catheter: Small tube used to remove mucus from the infant's nose, throat, or trachea to help maintain a clear breathing passage.

Synchronizer: A small soft circle attached to the abdomen. It is used only with certain kinds of respirators. It monitors the infant's initiation of inspiration so that the respiratory cycle can be in synchrony with the infant's breaths.

Temperature probe: A coated wire that detects temperature. This information regulates the amount of heat from the overhead heater or isolette.

Transcutaneous blood oxygen and/or carbon dioxide monitor: A noninvasive device that enables the reading of body oxygen levels and carbon dioxide through a sensor that attaches at the skin. This technique does not require the withdrawal of blood. This oxygen measurement is different from that of the pulse oximeter, so the numbers are different, usually lower.

Umbilical artery catheter (UAC) or umbilical venous catheter (UVC): Small piece of tubing threaded into the infant's artery or vein in the umbilical stump. In addition to delivering fluids, medication, and nutrients, blood can be withdrawn for lab work.

Warmer: A warmer is a bed that helps keep the infant's temperature stabilized.

Sources: Adapted from Mason (1994), Merenstein and Gardner (1985).

SECTION

MEDICAL DISORDERS AND OTHER ETIOLOGIES OF PEDIATRIC DYSPHAGIA

● ●

This section summarizes the major etiologies of pediatric dysphagia. The title of the topic is presented along with a description of the disorder. Clinical symptoms are listed as well as current medical intervention. Finally, a short summary of a typical treatment plan is presented under the heading "What Can We Do?" Details of specific therapy guidelines are presented in Section 5.

GASTROINTESTINAL/GASTROESOPHAGEAL TRACT DISORDERS

Many disorders can disrupt the successful digestion of food and ultimately infant feeding. Children with normal oral motor skills and swallowing function may have gastrointestinal (GI) issues that affect feeding. They will often refuse or be unable to tolerate oral feedings because of the negative consequences (i.e., respiratory distress, pain) associated with moving food from the esophagus to the intestines. This section summarizes some of the common GI disorders affecting children with swallowing/feeding problems.

Vascular Ring

Description

Vascular ring refers to a variety of anomalies of the aortic notch in which a "ring" of vessels surround the trachea, esophagus, or both, causing compression/obstruction (Gomella, Cunningham, & Eyal, 1994). Vascular rings are diagnosed early in infants; however, vascular anomalies that cause dysphagia have been reported in older children (Kosko, Moser, Erhart, & Tunkel, 1998).

Clinical Symptoms/Diagnosis

The infant presents with clinical signs of respiratory distress that worsens when eating, which in turn causes dysphagia. Diagnosis of this condition has been historically done with angiography (Kosko et al., 1998). With advances in imaging techniques, vascular rings now can be confirmed with a videofluoroscopic swallow study (to rule out aspiration) and esophagram (Gomella et al.,1994). Enhanced Computerized tomography (CT) or magnetic resonance imaging (MRI) is also used (Kosko et al., 1998).

Treatment Summary

Surgical treatment is recommended for severe cases. Surgery consists of division or suspension of the vessel (Kosko et al., 1998).

Tracheoesophageal Fistula/Esophageal Atresia

Description

In tracheoesophageal fistula (TEF) there is a communication between the esophageal and tracheal wall. Congenital TEF is caused by failure of the laryngotracheal tube to successfully separate from the esophagus during the embryonic period of neonatal development. This results in a variety of anomalies that can occur with esophageal atresia (EA). One classification of TEF/EA is presented in Figure 2–1. In EA, the upper two thirds (proximal end) of the esophagus ends about 10 centimeters (cm) from the nasopharynx in a completely closed pouch. EA can occur with or without TEF. In the majority of cases (85%), the distal esophagus is connected to the trachea (C-type TEF). Atresia alone occurs in only about 7% of the population (Gomella et al.,1994; Kosko et al., 1998). Together, tracheoesophageal/esophageal atresia constitute the most common congenital abnormality (Kosko et al., 1998). TEF also may be acquired through trauma (e.g., motor vehicle accident, intubation, tracheotomy).

Clinical Symptoms/Diagnosis

In TEF, liquids (formula or breast milk) enter the trachea during first feedings, causing the infant to choke, cough, gag, or become cyanotic and show other clinical

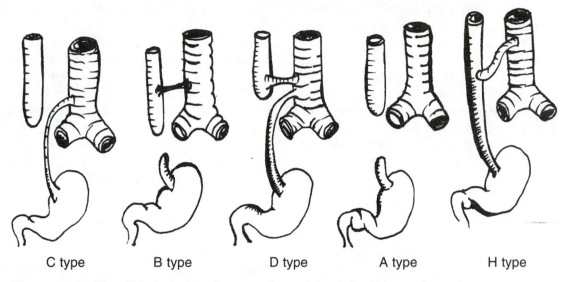

| C type | B type | D type | A type | H type |

Figure 2–1. Classification of tracheoesophageal fistula/esophageal atresia.

signs of respiratory distress. If TEF is accompanied with EA, the infant may vomit during the first feeding. Inability to place a nasogastric tube may trigger a consult for a videofluoroscopic swallow study (VFSS) with esophagram. Diagnosis of this condition is confirmed with a VFSS study (to rule out aspiration) with esophagram.

Treatment Summary

Surgical repair for all types of TEF/EA is required. The timing and extent of the repair depends on the classification. In some cases, esophageal reconstruction is necessary and can include grafts to lengthen the esophagus (i.e., colonic and jejunal grafts). The risk of morbidity increases with the length of the needed repair (Kosko et al., 1998). Surgical repair of TEF, and in some cases multiple repairs, can result in reduced esophageal motility during feeding.

Gastroesophageal Reflux

Description

Gastroesophageal reflux (GER) is the anterior return of the stomach contents into the esophagus and possibly the pharynx. Regurgitation or vomiting refers to the passage of stomach contents out of the mouth. Normal episodes of reflux can occur at least once per day in more than half of infants under the age of 3 months. Between 8 and 12 months, episodes of GER decrease dramatically (Nelson, Chen, Syniar, & Christoffell, 1997). GER can accompany many disorders seen in infants such as prematurity, cerebral palsy, incompetent lower esophageal sphinctor (LES), and gastrostomy tube placement (Boyle, 1989; Canal, Vane, Gotto, Gardner, & Grosfeld, 1987; Omari et al., 1998). Other etiologies include traumatic brain injury and nasogastric (NG) tube placement (Rossi, 1993). Children with a developmental disability often exhibit GER (Boyle, 1989). They may also show behavioral GER in which they gag, vomit, or ruminate stomach contents. In addition, poor posturing of high- and low-tone children can result in abdominal pressure that can push food into the esophagus through a normally functioning LES (Batshaw & Perret, 1995).

The amount of time its takes for the stomach to move food into the small intestine (gastric emptying) is also a factor in GER because this increases the time available for reflux to occur (Rossi, 1993). Left untreated, GER can lead to gastroesophageal reflux disease (GERD), which in turn can cause pneumonia, esophageal strictures, and esophagitis (Nelson et al., 1997). GER has been associated with Sandifer's sign (turning head to the left) laryngospasms, respiratory arrest, apnea, and apparent life-threatening events (ALTs) (Orenstein & Orenstein, 1988; See et al., 1989). Children with GER are at risk for failure to thrive (FTT), poor weight gain, and oral thrush.

Clinical Symptoms/Diagnosis

Children with GER may domonstrate projectile vomiting, coughing/choking, gagging, abnormal posturing (back arching), and/or irritability after feeding. Some infants may refuse feeding. Apnea and bradycardia (As and Bs) and hypoxemia may also be present (Gomella et al., 1994; See et al., 1989). Other airway complications that may be symptoms of GERD include frequent pneumonia, wheezing, reactive airway disease, stridor, and cough (Rudolph, 1997). Medical diagnosis is typically through a reflux scintiscan (scintigraphy) or pH probe examination. A barium swallow or esophageal endoscopy may offer information regarding the structural integrity of the esophagus.

Treatment Summary

Both medical and behavioral management are combined in the treatment of GER. Drug therapy typically includes medications to increase the resting tone of the LES, increase GI transit time (Reglan®, Bethanechol®, Propulsid®), and decrease gastric acid secretions (Tagamet®, Zantac®, and others). The side effects of these medications, fatigue, restlessness, and drowsiness, can affect feeding. By 18 months, most infants develop postural support, which usually results in a decrease of GER (Arvedson & Brodsky, 1993). Persistent GER or GER associated with G-tube placement may require surgery (Nissen fundoplication, Thal) to strengthen the tonicity of the LES.

ASSOCIATED FEEDING/SWALLOWING PROBLEMS

❖ Behavioral feeding problems/food and texture aversions

❖ Limited food repertoire, preference for thin liquids

❖ Aspiration (including aspiration of refluxed material)

❖ Emesis, rumination, reswallowing

❖ Crying, irritability, and fussiness during meals; back arching during/after feeds

❖ Coughing during feeds

❖ Snacking

❖ Sleep problems

❖ Episodic drooling

❖ Oral defensiveness/delayed feeding skills

WHAT CAN WE DO?

❖ Increase the caloric density and change the consistency. Thicken the liquids with dry cereal (1 tsp per ounce of formula or breast milk). This may not reduce the occurrence of GER, but it has been shown to decrease emesis (Orenstein et al., 1987; Rossi, 1993).

❖ Place the child at a 30° angle, prone upright position. Do this by elevating the head of the bed; do not use a car seat. This helps keep food away from the LES (Orenstein & Whitington, 1983; Rossi, 1993; Rudolph, 1997).

❖ Determine the optimal position. Keep the child quiet and in an upright, prone position for 30 minutes (or longer) after eating to allow for gastric emptying.

❖ Encourage NNS after meals.

❖ Decrease the volume of feeding and feed more frequently. In some cases of GERD associated with nonneurological or metobolic FTT, *increasing* the volume of feeding, even if vomiting occurs, may result in weight gain.

❖ Maintain nothing by mouth (NPO) 3 to 4 hours before bedtime.

Malabsorption Disorders of the Small Intestine

Description

Malabsorption disorders are caused by inadequate digestion and absorption of nutrients by the small intestine. The most common problems are *lactose intolerance* and *gastric dumping*.

Clinical Symptoms/Diagnosis

With lactose intolerance, the infant experiences emesis and possibly explosive diarrhea with abdominal bloating and gas after ingestion of milk or milk products (Batshaw & Perret, 1998). Infants with lactose intolerance may suffer failure to thrive (FTT) until they switch to a soy-based formula. Weight gain of less than 200 to 250 grams per week (6 to 8 oz) in infants less than age 4 months is inadequate (www.merck.com). To ensure weight gain, infants at risk for FTT are often placed on high calorie formulas or supplements, which then can lead to gastric dumping. Here, the stomach rapidly pushes inadequately digested food into the small intestine. This may cause abrupt changes in insulin levels, diarrhea, pallor, changes in pancreatic function, and/or sweating (Batshaw & Perret, 1998). Medical diagnosis is with a stool pH. A strong family history is usually present (Gomella et al., 1994).

Treatment Summary

Behavioral management is to avoid milk products and switch to soy-based products. Drug therapy can assist in breaking down the carbohydrates in milk before they reach the small intestine.

ASSOCIATED FEEDING/SWALLOWING PROBLEMS

❖ Behavioral feeding problems/food aversion.

WHAT CAN WE DO?

- ❖ Reduce oral aversion to feedings.
- ❖ Consult with a nutritionist/dietician to determine if a higher calorie formula would be tolerated.

Necrotizing Entercolitis/Short Gut Syndrome

Description

Necrotizing enterocolitis (NEC) is a serious intestinal disease caused by a combination of factors affecting the immature gut in premature infants. Ischemia or toxic damage weakens the mucosal lining of the intestinal walls. Bacteria then react to a substrate (breast milk or formula) followed by explosive bowel gas that leads to necrosis or gangrene of the bowel or bowel perforation. NEC primarily affects high-risk preterm infants (60–80%) but may also occur in full-term infants who have suffered acute cardiopulmonary distress or asphyxia (Gomella et al., 1994). NEC is classified into five stages ranging from suspected NEC (Stage 1) to advanced NEC (Stage IIIB).

Clinical Symptoms/Diagnosis

Symptoms of NEC occur after the infant's first oral or enteral feedings (3–7days). NEC is suspected if there is an intolerance to feedings, abdominal distention, bloody stools, episodes of As and Bs, and lethargy (Kliegman, 1990). Laboratory and radiographic studies confirm it.

Treatment Summary

The first course of medical treatment is strict NPO, bowel decompression, and antibiotic therapy. Feedings may be initiated in 3 days if the infant improves. For advanced NEC (Stages IIA and B), the infant will maintain NPO for at least 2 weeks with total parenteral nutrition (TPN). In cases where intestinal perforation occurs, surgical resection is required. *Short gut (or short bowel) syndrome* occurs when portions of the intestines are surgically removed. In addition to NEC, other conditions may result in short gut syndrome such as (a) intestinal malrotation (migration of the intestines into the abdominal wall with rotation of the small intestine), (b) midgut volvus (twisting of the small intestine causing obstruction), (c) intestinal atresias (failure of the development of part of the intestinal wall causing absence of a normal opening), and (d) abdominal wall defects (congenital herniation of the abdominal contents into the umbilical cord, known as omphalocele or beside the umbilical cord without a covering membrane, known as gastroschisis). Children with short gut syndrome receiving long-term TPN also receive oral or enteral feedings to help promote normal function of the remaining intestines (Rossi, 1993).

ASSOCIATE FEEDING/SWALLOWING PROBLEMS

- ❖ Behavioral feeding problems/food aversion.

WHAT CAN WE DO?

- ❖ Reduce oral aversion to feedings.

❖ Oral Motor: Maintain and promote the development of normal feeding skills.

RESPIRATORY DISORDERS

There are numerous conditions that can cause respiratory distress in infants. Any time breathing is compromised, feeding is affected. Typical causes of respiratory distress in newborn infants are anatomic, cardiac, and/or central nervous system (CNS)/peripheral nervous system (PNS) abnormalities. According to Arvedson (1998), there are several basic requirements that must be met before oral feeding can be attempted with any child, particularly medically fragile children:

❖ Cardiopulmonary stability

❖ Alert, calm stage

❖ In young infants, demonstration of rooting responses

❖ Adequate nonnutritive sucking

❖ Appetite or observable interest in eating

Description

Anatomic abnormalities of the oronasopharynx or larynx causing obstructive apnea:

1. *Choanal atresia:* A congenital disorder that affects 1 in 7,000 live births. The nasopharynx is blocked by either the nasal septum or soft tissue membrane. The infant is unable to breathe adequately through the nose. If there is complete obstruction, respiratory distress symptoms are immediate because of the infant's obligate nasal breathing. In this case, immediate airway intervention is needed. However, if there is partial blockage or stenosis, symptoms may only be present during feeding (Kosko et al., 1998). Most children with choanal atresia also present with other anomalies (Bergstrom & Owens, 1984).

2. *Midface hypoplasia:* A congenital disorder causing lack of development of the midfacial region. It is typically seen in Crouzon and Apert syndromes.

   ❖ *Hemifacial microsomia:* Lack of development of half of the face (Goldenhar syndrome)

3. *Mandibular hypoplasia:* The lack of development of the mandible that causes a normal size tongue to retract and obstruct the airway (glossoptysis). Typically seen in Pierre Robin sequence.

4. *Laryngeal anomalies:* Laryngeal abnormalities are often accompanied by respiratory compromise and can lead to dysphagia.

   ❖ *Laryngomalacia:* Failure of the cartilages of the larynx to harden. The larynx collapses during inspiration. Stridor during activity and crying are usually the first symptoms (Kosko et al., 1998). In cases of severe laryngomalacia, the infant is unable to tolerate the increased respiratory effort during feedings. If symptoms do not resolve by the first year, surgery (epiglottoplasty) may be required to maintain a patent airway (Zalzal, Anon, & Cotton, 1987).

❖ *Vocal fold paralysis:* Unilateral or bilateral damage to CN X (Vagus) or congenital anomalies cause the vocal folds to fail to completely open (abductor paralysis) or close (adductor paralysis). In abductor paralysis, the vocal folds are unable to open and may obstruct the airway. In adductor paralysis, they may fail to close completely during the swallowing. The deficient airway protection may lead to aspiration.

❖ *Laryngeal web:* Failure of the vocal folds to completely separate, leaving a thin "web" of muscosa attaching the two vocal folds (congenital). Acquired webs may be caused by laryngeal trauma such as oral intubation. Surgical resection is necessary.

❖ *Laryngotracheal cleft:* Rare congenital disorder in which the larynx and/or trachea fail to separate completely from the esophagus resulting in a communication between the larynx/trachea and esophagus. Depending on the degree of the cleft and subsequent aspiration, surgery is required. Laryngeal clefts are often associated with other congenital anomalies that also involve the gastrointestinal tract. For example, in Opitz G syndrome, the laryngeal cleft is accompanied by other midline defects including cleft palate, tracheoesophageal fistula, and hypospadias (congenital defect in which the urethra opens on the undersurface of the penis in males or into the vagina in females) (Kosko et al., 1998).

5. *Tracheoesophageal fistula* (see pp. 48–49)

6. *Apnea:* Cessation of breathing (respiratory gas flow) for longer than 20 seconds. Central apnea is caused by CNS problems and is characterized by no respiratory gas flow and no respiratory effort. Obstructive apnea is caused by anatomic/physiologic problems and is characterized by continual respiratory effort but no respiratory gas flow. Mixed apnea is a combination of central and obstructive apnea. Most commonly seen in premature infants, apnea may be caused by immaturity of the respiratory control mechanism, a response to hypoxia, sleep related (inability to shift from sleep to wakeful state), and muscle weakness. Apnea can accompany many disorders such as NEC, GERD, anemia, sepsis, and CNS disorders (Gomella et al., 1994)

Clinical Symptoms/Diagnosis

Children with respiratory disorders may demonstrate airway obstruction, respiratory stridor, changes in heart rate (tachycardia or bradycardia), changes in respiratory rate (tachypnea or apnea), reduced endurance and color changes during feedings, poor coordination of suck-swallow-breathe (coughing/choking), and short sucking bursts.

Treatment Summary

Management is individualized. For some disorders, immediate surgery is needed to open the airway. For other disorders, therapeutic intervention is needed until the infant grows out of it (laryngomalacia). Regardless, the first objective of management is treating the underlying respiratory disorder. Medical management may include supplemental oxygen, continuous positive air pressure (CPAP), and/or pharmacologic therapy (theophyline, caffeine, and doxapram).

By far the greatest consequence of reduced respiratory function is an increase in the work load to breathe. Because respiratory compromised infants need greater energy to breathe, their heart rates and breath rates increase, which ultimately causes them to expend more calories. During feedings, their work load to breathe increases even more, and they subsequently fatigue early or exhibit "poor endurance" and can actually lose calories during a feeding instead of gaining weight (Harrison, 1983). Careful monitoring of an infant's physiologic function before, during, and after feeding is necessary.

General guidelines for monitoring physiologic function are:

❖ Begin by looking at the infant and assess the resting heart rate (HR), respiratory rate (RR), and oxygen saturation level (O2 sats).

❖ Determine monitor alarm parameters. Medical staff set the monitors for highs/lows (e.g., if rates go above or below a specified level, an alarm will be triggered). Typical monitor parameters are:

> HR: between 80 and 220
>
> RR: between 30 and 80–90
>
> O2 sats: do not go below 85.

❖ For most infants, the resting heart rate should be between 120–150. If the HR is above 160 check with the medical staff, especially if it jumps when you stimulate the infant.

❖ For most infants, RR should be between 30–65. Infants are rarely fed orally if the RR is 70 or above.

❖ For most infants, O2 sats should be above 95%. If the O2 sats are around 90 and the child is on a nasal canula (oxygen therapy), ask the medical staff if oxygen can be increased until the O2 sats reach 95% before you begin feeding.

❖ Stop feeding the infant if any of these vitals change dramatically with presentation of the bottle or if the monitors go off. Usually, these changes mean the infant cannot handle feeding and needs more time.

ASSOCIATED FEEDING/SWALLOWING PROBLEMS

❖ Reduced endurance

❖ Uncoordinated suck-swallow-breathe sequence

❖ Weak suck

❖ Number of sucks per swallow increases as feeding increases

❖ Agitation during feedings

WHAT CAN WE DO?:

- ❖ Do not attempt to nipple feed children whose resting respiratory rate is above 70 breaths per minute (BPM) (Wolf & Glass, 1992).

- ❖ Monitor all physiologic functions (heart and respiratory rate) to determine the infant's tolerance to the feeding. Consult with the physician and/or nurse to determine if oxygen support can be increased during feedings. Some infants with "adequate" saturation levels may benefit from supplemental oxygen support during nipple feeding (Wolf & Glass, 1992).

- ❖ External pacing

- ❖ Consult with the nutritionist/dietician to determine if a higher calorie formula would be tolerated.

CENTRAL NERVOUS SYSTEM DAMAGE

Trauma to the CNS causing dysphagia in children can occur before, during, and after birth. CNS damage is often accompanied by pervasive/widespread developmental delays, behavioral problems, and dysphagia. Cerebral palsy is one of the more common disorders caused by CNS damage (Batshaw & Perret, 1998). This section focuses on pediatric dysphagia as it relates to damage to the CNS that may result in cerebral palsy.

Causes of CNS damage in children include:

- ❖ Cerebrovascular accident (intracranial hemorrhage)

- ❖ Traumatic brain injury (TBI)

- ❖ Neurologic diseases (encephalopathy, neural tube defects, tumors)

Other examples of neurologically based feeding disorders are summarized in Table 2–1.

Intracranial Hemorrhage

Description

Intracranial hemorrhage (ICH) is a descriptive term to indicate rupture of a blood vessel within the brain, brain stem, and cerebellum. ICH is common in preterm infants weighing less that 1500 grams and may also occur in infants suffering birth asphyxia and/or respiratory distress syndrome. One type of ICH predominatly seen in premature infants is intraventricular hemorrhage (IVH). In IVH, blood vessels surrounding the ventricles hemorrhage because of the difficulty the premature brain has managing blood pressure changes. IVH has been traditionally classified from Grade 1 to Grade 4, describing severity based on the location and size of the ventricles. In Grade 3, the bleeding into the ventricles is so great that the child may need to have the cerebral spinal fluid drained daily (a.k.a. reservoir) using needle aspiration through a very small opening through the skull. This procedure is different from a shunt. Over 75% of infants with Grade 3 IVH demonstrate significant developmental delays (Gomella et al., 1994).

TABLE 2–1. Neurologic Conditions of Childhood Associated With Feeding Disorders

A. Diffuse or bilateral dysfunction of cortex or basal ganglia
1. Static encephalopathy with neuromotor deficits
   a. *Prenatal onset:* brain dysgenesis, in utero intoxications, chromosomal defects, cerebrovascular accidents
   b. *Perinatal onset:* hypoxia-ischemia, hypoglycemia, complicated prematurity, CNS infection, cerebrovascular accidents
   c. *Postnatal onset:* trauma, hypoxia-ischemia, CNS infection, hypoglycemia, intoxications, cerebrovascular accidents
2. Progressive encephalopathy with neuromotor deficits
   a. *Metabolic:* inborn errors of metabolism, Wilson's disease
   b. *Infectious/postinfectious:* SSPE, HIV
   c. *Demyelinating:* multiple sclerosis
   d. *Other:* juvenile Huntington's, Pelizeus-Merzbacher, postirradiation, vasculitis, drug-induced movement disorders (neuroleptics, dilantin, reglan)

B. Brain stem
1. *Congenital CNS anomalies:* Arnold-Chiari malformation, syringomyelia, Mobius anomaly, congenital varicella infection
2. *Skeletal dysplasias:* dwarfism with foramen magnum stenosis, osteopetrosis, some craniosynostoses
3. *Malignancy:* tumors of the brain stem or posterior fossa
4. *Metabolic:* mitochondrial encephalomyopathy
5. *Trauma:* diffuse axonal injury
6. *Vascular:* cerebrovascular accident, arteriovenous malformations
7. *Infection:* brain stem encephalitis
8. *Demyelinating:* multiple sclerosis

C. Cranial nerves
1. *Trauma:* basilar skull fracture
2. *Motor neuron disease:* spinal muscular atrophy, poliomyelitis, juvenile amyotrophic lateral sclerosis, progressive bulbar paralysis of childhood, facioscapulohumeral neurogenic atrophy, congenital hypomyelination neuropathy
3. *Tumors:* schwannoma (neurofibromatosis)
4. *Demyelinating:* Guillian-Barré syndrome (acute and chronic)
5. *Toxins:* diphtheria, heavy metals

D. Neuromuscular junction
1. Myasthenia gravis
2. *Drugs/Intoxications:* botulism, organophosphate poisoning, tetanus, streptomycin, neomycin, kanamycin, bacitracin, polymyxin, colistin, Mg, beta blockers, phenothiazines, trimethaphan, methoxyflurane

E. Muscle
1. *Congenital:* myotonic dystrophy, congenital muscular dystrophy, congenital myopathies
2. *Inflammatory:* dermatomyositis, polymyositis
3. *Familial or metabolic:* facioscapulohumeral dystrophy, mitochondrial encephalomyopathy, ocular muscular dystrophy, inborn errors of metabolism affecting muscle
4. *Endocrine:* hyper- and hypothyroidism; steroid myopathy

F. Esophageal motility
1. *Associated with CNS dysfunction:* incoordination of pharyngeal and esophageal phases of swallowing, deficient central regulation of esophageal peristalsis
2. Induced by reflux esophagitis
3. *Drug-induced:* beta adrenergics, anticholinergics, muscle relaxants
4. Associated with myopathies

Source: From Ichord, R. (1994). Neurology of deglutition. In D. Tuchman and R. Walter (Eds.), *Disorders of feeding and swallowing in infants and children: Pathophysiology, diagnosis, and treatment* (p. 42). San Diego: Singular Publishing Group. Reprinted with permission.

Clinical Symptoms/Diagnosis

Infants with ICH may show changes in muscle tone, consciousness, and seizure activity. ICH may be asymptomatic and must be confirmed with head CT. Severe bleeding into the ventricles can cause an infant's hematocrit to drop, fontanels to bulge, and seizures to occur. Infants with small bleeds may recover neurologically. More severe hemorrhages may lead to hydrocephalus or porencephalitc cysts, a cavity within the cerebrum that opens into a ventricle. If a blood vessel bursts releasing blood under pressure, this can cause the cerebral tissue to tear. In addition, ischemia to the surrounding tissue can lead to cerebral infarcts (death of brain tissue caused by loss of blood). These children are likely to have abnormal unilateral muscle tone (hyper- or hypotonia) and cerebral palsy (Batshaw & Perret, 1998). Medical management includes maintaining arterial blood pressure and blood volume, drug therapy to increase production of cerebrospinal fluid, and placement of a ventricular drain or shunt (Gomella et al., 1994). Feedings are typically not initiated until the preterm infant is neurologically and medically stable. Wolf and Glass (1992) note that infants with severe ICH may not present with feeding problems once they are medically stable. Older children with developmental delays and cerebral palsy may exhibit motor-based feeding problems.

Traumatic Brain Injury

Description

Traumatic brain injury (TBI) is the most common cause of acquired disabilities in children (Finlayson & Garner, 1994). Common causes of TBI in infants are falls, motor vehicle accidents (MVA), and assault (i.e., shaken-baby syndrome). TBIs are broadly classified as penetrating (skull is perforated) or nonpenetrating (closed-head injuries). Nonaccelerating injuries occur when an object strikes a nonmoving head. This causes focal damage to the cortex (and meninges) at the site of impact and may result in blood clots, contusions, hemorrhages (epidural, subdural, subarachnoid, and/or intracerebral hematomas), cerebral edema, and ischemia. Acceleration injuries occur when the moving head contacts a nonmoving object. Shaken-baby syndrome is considered an acceleration injury because the brain damage occurs when the cranium strikes the skull (Brookshire, 1997). Acceleration injuries may cause diffuse lesions throughout the brain (nerve-cell axons) because of the twisting/torking and shearing/tearing forces. This condition, called diffuse axonal injury (DAI), often results in mild-severe communication, cognition, motor/sensory, and behavioral problems. Severe TBI can cause abnormal posturing. Decorticate posture (rigidity) results from diffuse white matter, thalamic, and internal capsule damage (mesencephalic region) and is characterized by flexion of the upper limbs that are drawn inward toward the shoulders. Decerebrate posture (rigidity) results from brain stem compression and is characterized by extension and internal rotation of the arms that are drawn to midline. The legs are extended and rotated inward with the feet flexed upward (forced plantar flexion) (Anderson & Anderson, 1990). In the most severe cases of TBI, the child remains in a persistent vegetative stage (Batshaw & Perret, 1998).

Clinical Symptoms/Diagnosis

Children suffering TBI without loss of consciousness may experience lethargy, irritability, initial vomiting, confusion, severe headaches, or changes in speech, motor movements, and vision. More severe injuries are followed by a period of deep, prolonged unconsciousness (i.e., coma) that may last minutes to years. The length and depth of the coma are correlated with the degree of brain injury and are measured using observational scales such as The Glasgow Coma Scale (Teasdale & Jennett, 1981) or the Comprehensive Level of Consciousness Scale (Stanczak et al., 1984). Medical management includes:

❖ Establishing medical stability (i.e., stopping hemorrhages and aiding respiration and blood pressure) to prevent secondary brain damage.

❖ Neurosurgery to remove blood clots, repair skull fractures, and relieve intracranial pressure.

Neurologic Diseases

Encephalopathy is acute or chronic damage to the cerebrum that may be caused by perinatal asphyxia (hypoxic encephalopathy), infection (encephalitis), severe jaundice (bilirubin encephalopathy), or congenital degenerative diseases (e.g., Leigh's disease, Schilder's disease).

Clinical Symptoms/Diagnosis

The amount of cognitive and physical deficits depends on the degree of brain tissue damage. Infants suffering from hypoxic encephalopathy at birth demonstrate low Apgar scores (0–3) for more than 5 minutes, seizures, and motor dysfunction (hypotonia). Infant states range from hyperalert-hyperreflexia to lethary-hyporeflexia. Some infants suffering from severe encephalopathy remain in a persistent vegetative state (David, Gomez, & Okazaki, 1970; Gomella et al., 1994).

Neural tube defects (NTDs) refer to a group of congenital anomalies that are caused by disruption of the developing brain and spinal cord. Spina bifida is the common term used to describe various neural tube defects. Classified as open or closed lesions, they can range from a small skin-covered sac along the vertebral column containing the meninges and cerebrospinal fluid (myelocele) to failure of anterior neural tube closure resulting in exposure of the degenerated brain outside of the cranium (anencephaly). Herniation of the spinal cord into a sac is called a myelomeningocele. Twenty-five percent of children with myelomeningocele are born with hydrocephalus (excessive accumulation of cerebrospinal fluid in the ventricles), a condition that can lead to severe neurologic involvement. Spina bifida aperta refers to a visible or open spinal cord defect (also called spina bifida cystica), whereas apina bifida occulta refers to hidden or nonvisible defects (www.sbaa.org).

Clinical Symptoms/Diagnosis

The degree of neurologic dysfunction depends on where along the spinal cord the lesion occurs. Higher lesions result in more severely impaired ambulation than lower lesions (Batshaw & Perret, 1998). Other complications of spina bifida include scoliosis; hip dislocation; paraplegia based on level of lesion; and sensory deficits in touch, pain, temperature, vibration, proprioception, and kinesthesia. All infants with anencephaly are stillborn or die within the first 2 weeks. In spina bifida with or without myelomeningocele, motor and sensory loss occurs below the site of lesion.

Tumors, either malignant or benign, can invade the brain or brain stem causing dysphagia. Most brain tumors in children (e.g., medulloblastoma, cerebellar astrocytoma, ependymomas) develop in the posterior fossa, the lower region of the brain. Tumors of the cerebral hemispheres (e.g., gliomas, craniopharyngioma) account for approximately 30% of pediatric brain tumors.

Clinical Symptoms/Diagnosis

Brain tumors may be difficult to diagnose because their symptoms can mimic other disorders. The symptoms also vary depending on the site of the tumor. Typical signs of brain tumors in infants include vomiting, seizures, drowsiness, increased head size, unexplained FTT, and dsyphagia (Rogers & Campbell, 1993; www.cbtf.org).

ASSOCIATED FEEDING/SWALLOWING PROBLEMS FOR CHILDREN WITH CEREBRAL PALSY

❖ Weak suck

❖ FTT

❖ Oral-motor instability caused by postural problems (i.e., hypotonicity, hypertonicity)

❖ Long-term enteral feedings

❖ Behavioral feeding problems (sensory-based feeding problems such as rumination, food/texture aversions, etc.)

WHAT CAN WE DO?

❖ Determine the optimal position. Treatment must be individualized to maximize posture, tone, and positioning for feeding hypertonic or hypotonic infants/children; semireclining position with 90° angle of the trunk and legs.

❖ Organize the infant for oral feedings.

❖ Consult with the nutritionist/dietician to determine if a higher calorie formula would be tolerated.

❖ Utilize a behavioral management program.

❖ Transition from tube feeding to oral feedings.

❖ Establish an optimal infant state: alter environment, alerting/calming cues, swaddle the infant.

❖ Oral motor: Maintain and promote the development of normal feeding skills.

❖ Reduce oral aversion to feeding.

❖ Alter consistency, temperature, and presentation of food.

PERIPHERAL NERVOUS SYSTEM DAMAGE

Congenital Myopathies/Muscular Dystrophy

Description

There are many different diseases that affect muscle. Congenital myopathies and muscular dystrophy refer to groups of muscle diseases that cause hypotonia and weakness that, in turn, affect respiration, feeding development, and swallowing. Although the progression is slow, most children with diseases of the muscle, particularly muscular dystrophy, do not live to adulthood (www.mda.org).

Clinical Symptoms/Diagnosis

Common symptoms include:

- ❖ Generalized weakness and atrophy of trunk and limb muscles, difficulty with postural control (e.g., Duchenne muscular dystrophy, congenital muscular dystrophy)

- ❖ Weakness and atrophy of shoulder, upper arm, and shin muscles with joint deformities (e.g., Emery-Dreifuss muscular dystrophy)

- ❖ Facial muscle weakness with atrophy of shoulders and upper arms (e.g., facioscapulohumeral muscular dystrophy)

- ❖ Weakness of the eyelid and pharyngeal constrictor muscles (e.g., oculopharyngeal muscular dystrophy)

- ❖ Generalized muscle weakness, weak cry, difficulty coordinating suck-swallow-breathe sequence (e.g., infantile progressive spinal muscular atrophy)

ASSOCIATED FEEDING/SWALLOWING PROBLEMS

- ❖ Weak suck
- ❖ Jaw clenching
- ❖ Reduced lip seal
- ❖ Tongue retraction, flat tongue with no central groove
- ❖ Reduced jaw/tongue movements or exaggerated jaw movements
- ❖ Poor coordination of suck-swallow-breathe sequence
- ❖ Early fatigue
- ❖ Difficulty with bolus preparation

WHAT CAN WE DO?

- ❖ Alter the nipple: liquid flow rate and stiffness
- ❖ Oral motor: maintain and promote the development of normal feeding skills and establish central tongue groove.
- ❖ Oral stimulation
- ❖ Establish optimal infant state: calming/alerting cues
- ❖ Alter the environment.
- ❖ Determine the optimal position: external postural support to ensure head, neck, trunk alignment
- ❖ Jaw and cheek support

CARDIAC DEFECTS

Respiration and Cardiac Systems

Description

The relationship between the respiratory and cardiac systems is reciprocal. Increases in cardiac demands cause an increase in the work load to breathe. There are many cardiac defects that affect infants and children. The consequence of these defects on respiration often leads to dsyphagia. The following are some of the more common pediatric cardiac anomalies.

Congenital heart disease (CHD): This is a generic term used to identify any malformations of the cardiovascular system in infants. CHD causes neonatal stress and is the most common cause of death, second only to complications of prematurity (Anderson & Anderson, 1990). Although usually identified at the time of birth, CHD may not be evident until weeks or years later.

Atrioventricular septal defect (AVSD): A malformation of the heart that results from failure of the normal separation of the ventricular inlet. This heart defect is a characteristic feature of Down syndrome and is seen in other syndromes. Untreated, it can lead to congestive heart failure.

Congestive heart failure (CHF): An abnormal condition of the heart caused by circulatory stress and congestion. In infants, CHF may be caused by stress to the heart from an overload of fluid and edema.

Patent ductus arteriosus: The ductus arteriosus is a duct that is open and used to bypass the lungs in the fetus. If the duct remains open after birth, oxygenated blood from the aorta flows into the pulmonary artery and then returns to the lungs. If left untreated (medication or surgery), a left to right shunt may develop, creating a pulmonary overload to the left side of the heart that can lead to CHF.

Tetralogy of Fallot: This heart defect is a result of four anomalies: pulmonary stenosis, ventricular septal defect, overriding aorta, and right ventricular hypertrophy. It causes deoxygenated blood to mix with oxygenated blood, reducing the amount of oxygenated blood sent out to the body.

Transposition of great arteries: The aorta and the pulmonary artery are attached to the incorrect ventricles, resulting in unoxygenated blood being carried to the body and oxygenated blood being carried to the lungs. If this occurs without other heart defects such as patent ductus arteriosus that would allow the oxyngenated and unoxygenated blood to mix, the infant dies within minutes of birth.

Coarctation of aorta: Narrowing of the aorta results in increased pumping of the left ventricle. This situation, in turn, causes increased blood pressure below the narrowing and decreased blood pressure below it.

Pulmonary stenosis: The valve or tissue between the right ventricle and the pulmonary artery is narrowed, decreasing the amount of unoxygenated blood reaching the lungs (Anderson & Anderson, 1990; Gomella et al., 1994).

ASSOCIATED FEEDING/SWALLOWING PROBLEMS

❖ Decreased endurance

❖ FTT

❖ Poor coordination of suck-swallow-breathe sequence

❖ Suck(le) lag, difficulty establishing a rhythmical suck(l)ing pattern

❖ As and Bs during feedings

❖ Oral defensiveness/sensitivity

WHAT CAN WE DO?

❖ External pacing

❖ Establish rhythmical NNS.

❖ Establish an optimal infant state: calming/alerting cues; external rhythm

❖ Monitor physiologic function: HR, RR, and O2 sat paramaters are dictated by the cardiologist. Typically, the O2 sat levels for infants with cardiac problems are kept down so that they hover around 85–90 to avoid over-working the heart.

❖ Reduce oral aversion to feeding.

❖ Establish an appropriate feeding schedule in collaboration with the pediatric nutritionist and physician.

EXTRACORPOREAL MEMBRANEOUS OXYGENATION

Description

Extracorporeal membraneous oxygenation (ECMO) is a highly invasive technique designed to provide temporary life support in infants more than 34 weeks gestation who are suffering from severe respiratory failure caused by meconium aspiration, pneumonia/sepsis, congenital diaphragmatic hernia, persistent pulmonary hypertension, asphyxia, hypoxia, hypercapnia, and/or acidosis. ECMO provides an external means of respiratory and cardiac support, thereby allowing the lungs to heal. Blood from the internal jugular vein and common carotid are distributed to the ECMO unit, oxygenated, rewarmed, and returned to the aorta. As lung function improves, extracorporeal blood flow is reduced and more blood is allowed to pass through the lungs until the infant can eventually be removed from ECMO (Kanter, 1994).

ECMO can save the lives of some very critical newborn infants who would not otherwise survive with conventional therapy. However, the risks, long-term costs, and benefits of this technique are still being explored. Children who are treated with ECMO may exhibit normal to severe neurodevelopmental delay. One efficacy study showed that 71% of infants who were treated with ECMO and survived had normal cognitive and physical functions (UK ECMO Collaborative Trial Group, 1996).

Clinical Symptoms/Diagnosis

Infants requiring ECMO treatment are very sick and can present with a wide array of medical symptoms. Because the purpose of ECMO is to allow the lungs to heal, infants receive primary enteral feedings, and there is a general "hands-off" attitude among the nursing staff and physicians until the infant's medical condition improves. Once the infant can be weaned from ECMO, bottle feedings are usually attempted.

ASSOCIATED FEEDING/SWALLOWING PROBLEMS

- ❖ Oral defensiveness
- ❖ Poor coordination of suck-swallow-breathe sequence
- ❖ Poor endurance
- ❖ Weak suck

WHAT CAN WE DO?

- ❖ Oral stimulation
- ❖ Establish rhythmical NNS.
- ❖ External pacing
- ❖ Establish an optimal infant state: calming/alerting cues, external rhythm.
- ❖ Monitor physiology during meals.
- ❖ Establish an appropriate feeding schedule.

PREMATURITY

The health of a newborn infant is primarily affected by the gestational age (postconceptional age [PCA]) at birth and birth weight. Of the approximately 4 million live births per year, approximately 250,000 are premature births. Of these, 75,000 are born more that 6 weeks early (www.neonatology.org). Infants may be born full term (37–41 weeks) but small for their gestational age (SGA). An SGA infant by definition weighs two standard deviations below the mean weight for gestational age or below the 10th percentile for the gestational age (Gomella et al., 1994). Prematurity, on the other hand, refers to infants born before 37 weeks postconception age. A premature infant who is born at 30 weeks PCA and weighs 1350 grams would not be considered SGA because we would expect an infant at 30 weeks to weigh about 3 lbs (Battaglia & Lubchenco, 1967). The average full-term infant (38 weeks PCA) would be expected to weigh about 3000 grams (Harrison & Kositsky, 1983). Preterm and SGA infants are classified according to their weight at birth into three broad categories:

1. Low birth weight (LBW) infants weigh less than 1500 grams.
2. Very low birth weight (VLBW) infants weigh less than 1000 grams.
3. Extremely low birth weight (ELBW) infants weigh less than 800 grams.

A premature infant is *not* a smaller version of a full-term infant. Although all of the anatomic structures are in place, the preterm infant has significantly reduced body fat and immature lungs that often require ventilation. Their underdeveloped sensorimotor and neurologic systems are not designed to manage the extrauterine environment (see stages of alertness pp. 5, 8, 9). Thus, a preterm infant differs from a full-term infant in both appearance and behavior.

Pre-Term Infant (<36 weeks)	**Full-Term Infant**
Soles of feet are smooth, only one transverse crease	Soles of feet are covered with creases
Earlobe: shapeless, no cartilage	*Earlobe:* stiff, thick cartilage
Hair: fine, fuzzy, clumped together	*Hair:* course, silky
No muscle tone; head, legs, arms dangle loosely away from body; head lags when pulled to sitting position	Increased muscle tone; limbs drawn toward chest; minimal head support
Skin: thick coat of white vernix when washed away reveals red, wrinkled folds of skin, hair	*Skin:* soft, smooth, pink-white
Genitals are exposed (girls), testicles are not yet descended (boys)	Genitals are covered (girls), testicles are descended (boys)
Sleeps more than 80–100% of the time	Sleeps about 75% of the time
No head-neck-trunk stability	Head-neck-trunk stability
Reduced or absent fat pads	Fat pad present
Neurologic immaturity	Neurologic maturity
Extensor pattern	Physiologic flexion
Hypotonic	Normal muscle tone
CNS cannot process stimuli from environment, limbs flail and jerk, startles easily	Can focus attention on environment, calm, more smooth gross motor movements

Premature and SGA infants are both at risk for medical complications, developmental disabilities, and feeding/swallowing problems. Premature infants are at greater risk for cerebral palsy, speech and language disorders, attention deficits, and learning disabilities. This risk increases in infants who are born at 20 to 25 weeks gestational age (extreme preterm infants). Approximately 50% of all extreme preterm infants who survive have some form of disability (Wood, Marlow, Costeloe, Gibson, & Wilkinson, 2000). Common medical complications of prematurity include GERD, IVH, and NEC. Other problems are described below.

Retinopathy of Prematurity

Description

Retinopathy is a consequence of prematurity and may be related to prolonged oxygen therapy. It is characterized by detachment of the retina and subsequent blindness.

Clinical Symptoms/Diagnosis

Most premature infants who were exposed to oxygen therapy or who were born before 30 weeks and weigh less than 1800 grams are seen by a pediatric ophthalmologist.

Treatment Summary

In some cases, cryosurgery can prevent complete retinal detachment. The speech-language pathologist (SLP) will work together with the vision specialist and the family to modify and adjust the infant's environment to accommodate the visual impairment.

Infant Respiratory Distress Syndrome

Description

Infant respiratory distress syndrome (IRDS) is a respiratory disorder that develops in the first hours of life in preterm infants, especially those infants born 32 weeks or earlier. The cause is a surfactant deficiency (lipoproteins that allow the exchange of gases in the alveoli and promote elasticity of pulmonary tissue). When the infant first begins to breathe, the alveoli open, then collapse, and stick together after each breath (atelectasis). This condition inhibits pulmonary gas exchange, increases the work load of respiration (e.g., respiratory rate increases), and leads to apnea with subsequent hypoxemia. Acute cases of IRDS may be referred to as hyaline membrane disease (HMD).

Clinical Symptoms/Diagnosis

Symptoms of acute hypoxemia are cyanosis, restlessness, stupor, coma, apnea, rapid breathing, and tachycardia then bradycardia. The infant attempts to compensate for these symptoms by increasing rate and effort of respiration. This attempt leads to increased oxygen demand and consumption, which in turn affects the coordination of suck/swallow/breathe, fatigue, and respiratory rates. Other symptoms of IRDS include:

❖ fatigue, grunting on expiration

❖ rapid breathing (more than 60 breaths per minute)

❖ chest retraction, nasal flaring

❖ reduced O_2 sat, peripheral edema

❖ increased acidosis (retention of CO_2)

❖ reduced circulation

Treatment Summary

The goals of medical management are to maintain fluids and temperature control and establish pulmonary blood-gas exchange. Surfactant therapy has greatly increased the survival rate of these infants (Berry, Abrahamowicz, & Usher, 1997). Depending on the severity of respiratory compromise, some infants may only receive oxygen therapy or continuous positive oxygen therapy delivered through two nasal cannulas (*Continuous Positive Air Pressure*). Other cases require mechanical ventilation using positive end expiration pressure (PEEP). The most severe cases require ventilatory strategies designed to enhance gas exchange in children with very low tidal volumes such as high-frequency jet ventilation.

Bronchopulmonary Dysplasia

Description

Bronchopulmonary dysplasia (BPD) is a broad term used to define chronic lung disease (CLD) of prematurity, and often these terms are synonymous. BPD is a pulmonary disease subsequent to ventilation and oxygen therapy. Most often, premature infants treated for IRDS are left with BPD. BPD begins with damage to lung tissue caused by surfactant deficiency, exposure to high-pressure ventilators, and high oxygen doses. The scarring of the lung tissue (bronchioles), which is permanent, results in pulmonary hypertension that can lead to heart problems. Infants requiring prolonged weaning from mechanical ventilation may require tracheostomy.

Clinical Symptoms/Diagnosis

The progression of IRDS to BPD may be gradual. The symptoms are similar with regard to respiratory fatigue and effort. Infants with BPD demonstrate nasal flaring, sternal retraction, tachycardia, and cyanosis. The subsequent tachypnea may create increased abdominal pressure leading to GER. Infants may appear "barrel-chested" because air gets trapped in the lungs and cannot be exhaled. Complications of BPD include infections of the lower airway, prolonged hospitalization, and rehospitalizations. Repeated ventilation can cause laryngeal trauma and increased airway resistance (edema, spasms, mucous).

Treatment Summary

Medical treatment goals are to prevent further lung tissue damage, establish unassisted pulmonary function, and assist the growth and development of the infant. Oxygen and/or ventilator support, drug therapy, fluid restriction, and careful monitoring of caloric intake accomplish these goals.

ASSOCIATED FEEDING/SWALLOWING PROBLEMS

- ❖ GER
- ❖ FTT (developmental delays)
- ❖ oral defensiveness/hypersensitivity caused by aggressive respiratory intervention and prolonged NPO status
- ❖ behavior problems
- ❖ increased and/or inconsistent jaw opening in response to oral stimulation
- ❖ arrhythmic movements of the jaw and tongue
- ❖ tongue protrusion
- ❖ increased lip retraction
- ❖ decreased lip seal

❖ difficulty expressing milk from the nipple because of decreased jaw stability

❖ infant state (irritability, poor alertness)

❖ disorganized behaviors, especially suckling

❖ poor endurance (early fatigue during feeds, unable to sustain suckling for longer than 2 minutes)

❖ poor coordination of suck/swallow/breath that can lead to bradycardia, tachypnea, desaturation, and aspiration

❖ tracheostomy: poor neck posture, loss of smell, reduced pharyngeal transit of the bolus, increasing the risk of aspiration, oral defensiveness.

WHEN ARE PREMATURE INFANTS READY TO FEED?

❖ The infant is considered medically stable.

❖ Postural control has improved and the infant can bring hands to his or her face and mouth.

❖ Cardiopulmonary stability: Respiration is stable (even, rhythmic breathing pattern; oxygen saturation is 95% or better).

❖ The infant is in appropriate state before feeding (calm, pink, alert, organized).

❖ The infant demonstrates a rhythmic NNS.

❖ Typically, premature infants are not ready to bottle or breast feed prior to 32 weeks. Ideally, they should start feeding around 33–34 weeks.

WHAT CAN WE DO?

❖ With medical clearance and in collaboration with the pediatric nutritionist, establish appropriate feeding schedules; schedule change of NG feeds so the baby feels hungry.

❖ In collaboration with other medical professionals, educate the feeder (parents, etc.) on how to monitor physical parameters before, during, and after meals.

❖ Reduce oral aversion to feeding.

❖ Use oral stimulation to help increase suckling.

❖ Establish/promote NNS prior to oral feeding. Encourage pacifiers during tube feedings.

❖ Utilize a behavioral management program: reinforce pleasurable experiences.

❖ Alter the environment.

❖ Establish the optimal infant state: alerting/calming cues; swaddle the infant.

❖ Watch for signs of infant stress (see Table 1–6 on p. 10).

❖ Organize the infant for oral feedings. Decrease your movements to help the infant stay organized.

❖ Establish the optimal position: flexion and head-neck-trunk support.

❖ Alter the nipple: change nipple size and flow rate. Find the "easiest" bottle/nipple system that allows the infant to suck and swallow liquid with the least effort. Do not completely fill the bottle. A full bottle adds pressure and increases the flow rate. Instead, hold the bottle horizontally with the liquid only filling half to three quarters of the nipple. Less fluid will help slow the flow, allowing the infant to take breaks as needed.

❖ External pacing

❖ With medical approval, consider increasing oxygen during feedings for infants who require, or who have required, oxygen due to respiratory compromise. This will allow the infant to concentrate on extablishing a mature suck rather than trying harder to breathe.

❖ Loosen the diaper to help with belly breathing.

❖ Do not force the bottle if the infant does not open her or his mouth when presented with the nipple.

❖ Consider alternating between tube and oral feeding. This will allow the infant to expend less energy and be more organized for oral feedings.

❖ Monitor the infant's daily schedule. Be aware of tests or other procedures the infant may have had and avoid feeding around these times when the infant is likely to be fatigued and possibly stressed.

STRUCTURAL ABNORMALITIES

Many children presenting with dysphagia suffer from genetic defects that disrupt normal physiologic/neurologic development and affect the anatomic structures of swallowing. For example, craniofacial anomalies such as cleft lip and palate accompany many genetic defects that, in turn, affect feeding. Other children who are born addicted to cocaine present unique feeding challenges. Table 2–2 summarizes the genetic syndromes with prominent dysphagia. The following section highlights some of the more prevalent genetic disorders with associated feeding/swallowing problems.

CHARGE Association

This acronym stands for coloboma (cleft of the iris of the eye), atresia of the nasal cavity, heart disease, retarded growth, genital abnormalities, and ear disorders including deafness. Feeding/swallowing disorders are related to respiratory compromise and reduced tolerance to feeding caused by heart problems. Developmental delays are also a source of feeding problems.

Chiari Malformations

Previously referred to as Arnold Chiari syndrome, this is a group of genetic defects that affect the posterior fossa anatomy (brain stem, cerebellum, fourth ventricle). The defects range in degree of severity from minor displacements of cerebellar tissue to defective or incomplete development of the cerebellum. The syndrome is classified as Chiari I–IV. In the Chiari type I malformation, the cerebellar tonsils and a small part of the medulla oblongata herniate through the foramen magnum. It is typically

TABLE 2–2. Genetic Syndromes With Prominent Dysphagia

Diagnoses	Anomalies	Neurodevelopmental Profile	Feeding Abnormalities
Prader-Willi	Narrow bifrontal diameter Almond-shaped palpebral fissures Small hands and feet Obesity	Mental retardation and hypotonia	Dysphagia frequently observed in the first year
Coffin siris	Microcephaly, growth deficiency Coarse facies, full lips, wide mouth Sparse scalp hair Hypoplastic or absent fifth digit	Mental retardation and hypotonia	Difficulty sucking, swallowing, and breathing
Oculo-mandibulo-facial syndrome (Hallerman Streiff)	Short stature (proportionate) Dyscephaly, frontal bossing Mandibular and nasal cartilage hypoplasia Microstomia, glossoptosis Microphthalmia Hypostrichosis	Normal intelligence	Feeding and respiratory problems are common during infancy
Freedman-Sheldon	Mask-like "whistling facies" Hypoplastic alae nasi Club feet	Hypotonia, facial paresis and possible myopathic arthrogryposis	Feeding problems secondary to severe microstomia
Smith-Lemli-Optiz syndrome	Microcephaly, narrow high forehead, prominent metopic suture Hypospadia, cryptorchidism Short nose, anteverted nose, ptosis Broad maxillary-alveolar ridge Syndactyly of second and third toes	Moderate to severe mental poor suck, retardation Hypotonia progressing to hypertonia	Gastroesophageal reflux
de Lange syndrome	Hirsutism, synophrys Microcephaly Thin down-turned upper lip Micomelia, oligodactyly, or phocomelia	Mild to severe mental retardation Spasticity, motor delays	Poor suck, frequent respiratory infections
Dubowitz	Low birth weight and postnatal growth retardation Microcephaly Hoarse cry Small facies, shallow nasal bridge, telecanthus, ptosis Micrognathia	Mild mental retardation common	Poor oral intake, frequent emesis and diarrhea during first year

Syndrome	Characteristics	Development	Feeding/Swallowing
Pierre Robin sequence	Mandibular hypoplasia Micrognathia U-shaped cleft palate	Generally normal development	Respiratory distress with feeding in infancy including coughing, grunting, and sputtering
Facioauriculo vertebral spectrum	First and second branchial arch anomalies Microtia Maxillary and mandibular hypoplasia	Normal development	Respiratory distress with feeding in infancy
Klippel-Feil	Short neck Low hairline Fusion of cervical vertebrae	Syringomelia may develop	Cranial nerve deficits result in dysphagia
Mobius sequence	"Mask-like" facies at birth Cranial nerve palsies	Cognitive development usually normal	Paralysis of cranial nerves VI and VII (usually permanent) Dysphagia not usually severe unless other cranial nerves involved (V, IX, X, or XII)
Rubenstein-Taybi	Short stature Downward slanting palpebral fissures Hypoplastic maxilla and narrow palate Broad thumbs and toes	Mental retardation Motor delays	Infants have a weak suck Swallowing is poorly coordinated Frequent vomiting during infancy
Beckwith-Wiedemann	Macroglossia Omphalocele Ear creases Macrosomia	Mild to moderate mental retardation has been reported Development can be normal	Feeding problems secondary to large tongue
Trisomy 18	Growth deficiency Prominent occiput Low-set ears Short sternum Congenital heart defects Micrognathia, narrow palate	Profound mental retardation Hypertonia	High-pitched cry Poor suck
Trisomy 21 (Down syndrome)	Brachycephaly with relatively flat occiput Upward slanting palpebral fissures Small nose with flat nasal bridge Small ears Short metacarpals and phalanges Single transverse palmar crease	Hypotonia Usually moderate mental retardation	Weak suck Feeding can be further compromised by cardiovascular anomalies

Source: From Arvedson, J., and Brodsky, L. (1993). Pediatric swallowing and feeding: Assessment and management. San Diego: Singular Publishing Group. Reprinted with permission.

identified in adults and is often associated with syringomyelia (a disease causing cavities in the grey matter adjacent to the central canal of the spinal cord. The cavities cause loss of the sense of pain and temperature and in severe cases can cause paralysis). The Chiari type II malformation, which involves herniation of the vermis and the fourth ventricle, is usually associated with hydrocephalus and neural tube defects. Cerebellar hypoplasia, brain stem displacement, and elongation of the fourth ventricle occur. It is typically identified early in infancy (McLone, D., 2000).

If the brain stem displacement affects CN X, the child will present with nasopharyngeal reflux during feeding, vocal fold paralysis causing stridor when feeding/crying, and reduced pharyngeal contraction during swallowing. Involvement of other cranial nerves important for feeding (V, VII, XII) will cause difficulty with oral-motor aspects of feeding, which can be an early indicator of Chiari malformation. Klein and Delaney (1994) suggest that any changes in feeding warrant a consultation with the physician, as they may indicate changes in the malformation (Klein & Delaney, 1994)

Moebius Sequence

Infants born with Moebius sequence have damage to the 6th and 7th cranial nerves that result in oculofacial paralysis and may present with total absence of facial expression. If other cranial nerves are damaged (V, IX, X, XII), they will also demonstrate significant oral and pharyngeal dysphagia.

Freedman-Sheldon

General hypotonia and facial paralysis coupled with a small mouth affecting feeding.

Pierre Robin Sequence

A U-shaped cleft palate may be present. Glossoptosis (downward displacement of the tongue) and micrognathia (abnormally small mandible usually resulting in a recessive, bird-like profile) cause respiratory-based feeding problems as well as oral dysphagia.

Fetal Alcohol Syndrome

Presenting symptoms include growth retardation (prenatal and/or postnatal), possible cleft palate, midface hypoplasia, thinned upper lip, developmental delay, central nervous system dysfunction, and hearing loss. This, in turn, delays the development of feeding skills.

Maternal Substance Abuse/Infant Withdrawl

Most infants born addicted to CNS stimulants (i.e., crack cocaine, methamphetamine) have state-related feeding problems. They are very irritable, fussy, disorganized, and easily distracted. Infants born addicted to CNS depressants (i.e., alcohol, barbiturates) have a very weak suck, poor endurance, and difficulty with suck-swallow-breathe sequence. Some infants who are hyperalert may demonstrate an exaggerated suck pattern with poor respiratory coordination.

What Can We Do?

❖ Establish optimal infant state: alter environment/calming cues.

❖ Determine optimal feeding position.

❖ Alter the nipple: Children with cleft palates and some oral motor problems caused by muscle weakness may benefit from a softer nipple (Klein & Delaney 1994). Experiment with different nipples and establish the safest flow rate.

❖ Organize the infant for oral feedings. Swaddle the infant, maintaining a stable midline position.

❖ Provide external assistance for lips and/or jaw during feeding.

❖ External pacing

❖ Consult with a nutritionist/dietician to determine if a higher calorie formula would be tolerated.

❖ Reduce oral aversion to feedings.

Acquired Immune Deficiency Syndrome

The number of pediatric acquired immune deficiency syndrome (AIDS) cases is increasing (Committee on Pediatric AIDS, 2000). Human immunodeficiency virus (HIV) infection in children occurs in utero or perinatally via maternal blood and secretions, including breast milk. Children who subsequently are diagnosed with AIDS are at risk for developmental delay, encephalopathy, neuromuscular disorders, esophagitis, and poor dentition (Layton & Davis-McFarland, 2000). Pressman and Morrison (1988) point out that these complications associated with AIDS may lead to nutritional compromise, reduced endurance for feeding, aspiration, social isolation, and failure to thrive.

ASSOCIATED FEEDING/SWALLOWING PROBLEMS

❖ Coughing/choking on thin liquids and solids

❖ Gagging

❖ Slow feeding

❖ Possible odynophagia (pain when swallowing)

❖ Hypersensitivity and oral defensiveness

WHAT CAN WE DO?

❖ Change the consistency: thicken liquids.

❖ Determine the optimal position.

❖ Avoid acidic foods/juices.

❖ Alter the food texture/temperature.

Nonorganic Failure To Thrive

Description

There are healthy children who present with long-term feeding problems in the absence of medical, motor, or cognitive deficits (nonorganic failure to thrive [NOFTT]). Typically, these children have a past history of serious medical conditions that required aggressive treatment and long-term stays in the NICU. Palmer and Heyman (1993) theorize that some premature and full-term infants, whose medical conditions have resolved and who present with normal oral-motor functioning, suffer from sensory-based oral feeding problems. These problems may or may not co-exist with behavioral feeding problems. Other children may present with behavioral feeding problems without a sensory component (generally stemming from a disordered feeding interaction or environmental or social problems).

Successful feeding interactions help the infant and young child develop and grow physically, help to develop cognitive and language skills, and are important for emotional development (Arvedson, 1998; Barnard, Hammond, & Booth, 1989). Regardless of etiology, it is generally believed that if a child fails to achieve normal feeding skills by 12 months of age, she or he is at risk for long-term feeding problems (Blackman & Nelson, 1985). Possible treatment goals for this population are:

❖ Maintain adequate nutrition and hydration.

❖ Practice aggressive nutritional and behavioral intervention.

❖ If the child is receiving primary enteral support, transition from tube to oral feedings.

❖ Attain age-appropriate feeding skills.

❖ Expand the food repertoire.

Clinical Symptoms/Diagnosis

These children often demonstrate poor growth and weight gain and typically fall into one of two groups of sensory-based feeding problems. The first group includes children with completely normal anatomy/physiology who present with a behavioral and/or psychologic feeding disorder. The second group includes children who have a behavioral and/or psychologic feeding disorder in the presence of neurological or anatomical involvement that may affect (or have affected) feeding development. However, their presenting symptoms are far more severe than can be explained by their physiology. The following are some examples of these two groups.

Sensory-Based Feeding Disorder: Normal Physiology

History of :
• Repeated orally invasive procedures
• GER
• GI disorders
• TEF
• Cardiac defects
• Respiratory disorders
• Autism
• Delayed introduction of oral feedings
• Prolonged use of orogastric (OG) or NG feeding
• History of multiple medical interventions
• History of force feedings

Sensory-Based Feeding Disorder: Abnormal Physiology

• Cerebral palsy
• Craniofacial anomalies
• Genetic defects

Regardless of etiology, the safety of swallowing (i.e., no aspiration and normal pharyngeal function) must be determined before initiating any treatment program. This determination typically includes a videofluoroscopic swallow study and is particularly important for children with histories of cardiac and/or respiratory compromise.

Children with nonorganic failure-to-thrive are a daily challenge for parents/caregivers at mealtimes. Parents/caregivers report that each meal is a "battle" that the child usually wins. If the child is able to achieve her or his expected weight/height goals, it is probably because she or he is snacking throughout the day rather than eating full meals. Children can display mild aversive behaviors such as food refusal or selectivity. More severe behaviors include extreme gagging and vomiting during meals. As is true for all children with feeding disorders, sensory-based feeding problems are highly individualized to the specific child. Some children will accept nonnutritive stimulation (i.e., mouthing fingers, toys, pacifiers), whereas others may not. Still others may present with mixed sensory responses, that is, they exhibit both hyper- and hyposensitivity (e.g., stuffing their mouths with food but with poor tactile discrimination to handle the food).

The following examples, adapted from Palmer and Heyman (1993), are indicators of a sensory-based versus motor-based oral feeding problem.

Motor-Based Problems

- *May* adapt to flow rate changes during feedings.

- Disorganized sucking may occur on any nipple type (trouble adapting to different flow rates).

- Feeds best in quiet-alert state.

- Will allow another's finger in mouth for nonnutritive sucking.

- Tolerates pureed and textured food better than liquids.

- Has difficulty with chewing.

- Gags only if swallow response is delayed or if aspiration occurs.

- Does not manage mixed food textures.

- Feeding problems are consistent but may worsen if the child is distracted.

Sensory-Based Problems

- Prefers one type of nipple and flow rate.

- Has nipple confusion.

- Feeds best when sleeping or woken from sleep (night-time feeding).

- May nonnutritively suck on thumb/finger/pacifier.

- Does not tolerate others touching her or his tongue or putting fingers in her or his mouth.

- Prefers liquids, especially water.

- Chews solids but holds food to avoid swallowing.

- Gags easily, especially when eating solids or when the spoon touches the lips.

- Separates and expels solid food pieces in mixed consistency foods.

- When distracted, swallows foods of different textures.

Treatment Summary

The key to successful feeding therapy is early identification of children at risk for NOFTT. Aggressive nutritional/behavioral interventions must be implemented early to reduce the effects of prolonged malnutrition and ensure successful child/caregiver interaction (Arvedson, 1998). Therapy should follow a sensory hierarchy that includes visual, olfactory, tactile, and gustatory interventions. A team approach to therapy will improve the chances for successful intervention. For example, collaboration with an occupational therapist specializing in sensory processing dysfunction is very helpful. In addition, behavioral feeding psychologists can implement a structured reinforcement program allowing the feeding therapist to do the therapy needed. Outpatient treatment approaches are presented in Section 4.

Therapy should begin in the least restrictive environment, preferably with a family-based treatment. Some parents may choose an intensive inpatient program. Here, successful treatment of NOFTT is contingent on the transition of successful feeding strategies to the nonhospital environment (Babbitt, Hoch, & Coe, 1994). Pharmocologic treatment coupled with a cognitive behavioral approach to therapy also has been attempted (Atkins, Lundy, & Pumariega, 1994).

SECTION

PROCEDURES

· ·

This section includes information pertinent to the assessment of children with dysphagia. This section begins with an overview of medically based diagnostic tests. Next, the various methods currently available for evaluation of swallowing function are described. Finally, indepth procedures for conducting a clinical assessment and videofluoroscopic evaluation of feeding/swallowing function are presented.

GENERAL DIAGNOSTIC PROCEDURES

The following diagnostic procedures were compiled from Berk (1995).

Gastroesophageal Reflux

An accurate diagnosis of gastroesophageal reflux (GER) in newborns involves the application of several tests. Often included are esophageal manometry, esophageal pH monitoring, scintigraphy, and videofluoroscopy. The goal, or purpose, of these procedures is twofold: (a) determine the quality of the musculature within the esophagus, particularly at the level of the lower esophageal sphincter (LES), and (b) determine the level of acidity within and above the level of the LES.

Esophageal Manometry (Esophageal Motility Study, Esophageal Function Study)

Esophageal manometry (EM) assesses the functional integrity of the esophageal musculature. Esophageal manometry is performed differently in children than in adults because of the size and maturation of the infant esopohagus and cooperation of the child. The procedure typically is completed within 15 minutes. A thin tube with openings is inserted nasally through the esophagus until part of the tube has entered the stomach. When this tube is positioned in the esophagus, the openings sense the pressure in various parts of the esophagus during a dry swallow elicited by a Santmyer swallow reflex or when the infant is swallowing small amounts of water. As the esophagus squeezes on the tube, these pressures are transmitted to a computer that records the pressures. Dynamic recordings of intraluminal pressure can also be made using a water-perfused tube. Here, the tube is inflated with water at various points creating a balloon-like shape. Once inflated, the resistance to the pressure by the esophageal musculature is calculated. EM cannot be used to diagnose gastroesophageal reflux alone. Rather it is one component of the total diagnostic procedure. For example, EM can help determine if further surgical intervention (i.e., fundoplication) is necessary to control GER. The procedure also is used to locate the LES for subsequent pH monitoring (American Gastroenterological Association, 1994; Clark, 1993; Kahrilas, Dent, Dodds, Hogan, & Arndorfer, 1987).

ADVANTAGES

1. EM can assess esophageal peristalsis during a swallow and the passive tension of the LES.

2. EM allows indirect observation of the cricopharyngeus muscle.

3. EM can be useful to locate the upper and lower esophageal sphincters for esophageal pH monitoring.

DISADVANTAGES

1. EM is not helpful in the medical management of gastroesophageal reflux disease or lesions of the esophagus.

2. Typically, EM must be combined with videofluoroscopy to visually identify the anatomical placement of the transducers.

3. EM is an invasive procedure and may not be tolerated well by children who are tactily defensive. Sedation may be necessary.

Esophageal pH Monitoring (Esophageal Probe)

The esophageal pH probe is the diagnostic procedure used to diagnose gastroesophageal reflux. In fact, it is considered to be the gold standard of GER diagnoses. A tube, often referred to as a probe, is inserted nasally and extended to a point a few centimeters above the LES. This point was identified by an earlier esophageal manometry study. The tube is left in place for 24 hours to fully quantify the transient levels of stomach acid found in the lower esophagus.

A pH level of 7.0 is considered neutral, whereas a pH level of < 4.5 is considered to be acidic. By leaving the probe in place for 24 hours, patterns of reflux activity can be recorded in terms of duration and intensity. Precipitating variables can be identified. The procedure is not indicated in patients who demonstrate obvious reflux. It typically is used to identify suspected trace reflux in newborns that is not necessarily behaviorally apparent. It can also be used with patients whose endoscopic evaluation appears normal, but whose symptoms indicate GER.

ADVANTAGES

1. The recording device is portable and can be used with active infants and children.

DISADVANTAGES

1. Esophageal pH monitoring is an invasive, long (24 hours) procedure.

Scintigraphy (Milk Scan or Technetium Scan)

Scintigraphy is an imaging technique used to examine the passage of radioactive material mixed in a liquid from the mouth through the stomach and is often used to calculate gastric emptying time. The radioisotope (technetium-99m pertechnitate) is either delivered to the stomach through a nasogastric (NG) tube or by ingestion. The infant is then scanned for 1–2 hours with a gamma camera to document evidence of reflux or gastric emptying time. The scan may also detect aspiration (occasionally), tracheoesophageal fistulas, esophageal atresia, and esophageal perforations.

ADVANTAGES

1. Scintigraphy can detect GER in instances where a pH probe does not (because of the nonacidic consistency of the refluxed material).

DISADVANTAGES

1. Scintigraphy is a long procedure (1–2 hours).
2. Radioactive material is used.

Barium Esophagram/Barium Swallow Test/Upper Gastrointestinal Series

This series is an x-ray test used to define the anatomy of the upper digestive tract. The patient is given liquid barium to drink, and the radiologist follows the barium fluoroscopically as it moves through and fills the esophagus, stomach, and duodenum (small intestine). Still x-ray films are taken. This test can reveal ulcers, tumors, hiatal hernias, scarring, blockages, muscular wall abnormalities, and so forth. A similar study, the air contrast esophagram, uses effervescent granules added to the barium to allow greater detailing of gastrointestinal anatomy. Because this test typically focuses on the anatomic structures of the esophagus, it is not the method of choice for evaluation of oral- or pharyngeal-based dysphagia.

ADVANTAGES

1. Barium esophagram/barium swallow test/upper gastrointestinal series test is a common test.
2. This test is good for evaluating esophageal anatomy and motility disorders.

DISADVANTAGES

1. Barium esophagram/barium swallow test/upper gastrointestinal series test uses radiation.

2. Although the test uses real-time fluorography, still x-ray films are taken; therefore, it does not provide a lasting record of the dynamics of swallowing.

Evaluation of Swallowing Function

The following evaluation procedures were compiled from Bastian (1998), Benson and Tuchman (1994), and Logemann (1998).

Ultrasoundography

A transducer is placed beneath the chin or on the cheek and is used to generate high-frequency sound waves (2–10 megahertz [MHz]) and to receive the echoes. Tissue contrast is provided by the differences in each tissue's ability to reflect sound. Air, water, and milk project as white; muscles, glands, and other soft tissue project as grey shades. Ultrasound echoes are then converted into a "real-time" image. New innovations are beginning to use color in the ultrasound image for easier identification. Although tongue movements during feeding are viewed best (Kramer & Eicher, 1993), the oropharynx can be viewed in babies and small children by angling the transducer (Benson & Tuchman, 1994).

ADVANTAGES

1. Ultrasoundography images may be obtained in sagittal, coronal, and transverse planes by rotating the transducer without moving the patient. The patient can be evaluated in an upright position, lying down, or sitting on a lap.

2. Images are collected in multiple planes in real time. Images can be frozen for immediate inspection, digitized and enlarged for further examination of fine details, or stored on videotape for later inspection.

3. Barium is not required: any amount or type of solid or liquid food can be imaged during swallowing.

4. Noninvasive: Ultrasoundography allows soft-tissue structures to be imaged that cannot be clearly defined using videofluorography.

5. Ultrasoundography can evaluate the effects of oral sensory motor stimulation techniques and study the sucking patterns of preterm infants.

6. Ultrasoundography is tyically used to assess the oral preparatory and oropharyngeal stages of swallowing (motion of the tongue and floor of mouth). It can be used repeatedly and for prolonged periods of time because there is no radiation exposure.

7. Portable: It can be used bedside or in an office.

8. Ultrasoundography is good for studying children with cerebral palsy or poor feeders who require frequent monitoring of the oral preparation and oral stages of deglutition.

DISADVANTAGES

1. Ultrasoundography cannot directly determine whether aspiration has occurred: the imaging field is not broad enough to view the mouth, pharynx, and esophagus simultaneously.

2. Soft areas behind the larynx and hyoid cannot be imaged.

3. Quality of images and interpretation depend on the operator.

4. Ultrasound will not pass through bone.

Fiberoptic Endoscopic Evaluation of Swallowing

Fiberoptic endoscopic evaluation of swallowing (FEES) is also known as videoendoscopic swallowing study (VESS). A flexible nasoendoscope is passed through the nose into the pharynx allowing visualization of the anatomical structures related to swallowing (palate, pharynx, tongue base, and larynx). Sensory testing of the superior laryngeal nerve is done by touching the tip of the endoscope to areas of the hypopharynx and larynx to assess the degree and symmetry of the reaction. Next, the patient swallows food and/or liquids mixed with methylene blue dye (Bastian, 1998) or green food coloring (Willging, 1995.) Videotape images of the pharynx and larynx can document premature spillage, laryngeal penetration, pharyngeal pooling, and residue (Willging, 1995).

Recently, more objective sensory testing has been combined with FEES, called fiberoptic endoscopic evaluation of swallowing with sensory testing (FEEST). Here, the endoscope is positioned 5 mm above the aeryepiglottic fold, and a small pulse of air is delivered. The threshold at which the pulse of air elicits vocal fold closure is measured. Bastian (1998) provides an excellent description of the procedures for videoendoscopic swallow study.

ADVANTAGES

1. FEES equipment is relatively inexpensive and portable.

2. It provides detailed information about pharyngeal and laryngeal structures.

3. It does not require the administration of food; therefore, it can be used to assess children with suspected vocal fold dysfunction or laryngotracheal abnormalities.

4. There is no radiation exposure, ingestion of barium, or time constraint.

5. It can be used to provide biofeedback as a part of swallowing therapy.

6. It is useful in assessing the patient's swallowing ability as well as the structures/function of swallowing before food is introduced.

7. It assists in assessing neurologic status and sensation.

DISADVANTAGES

1. FEES does not assess the oral or esophageal stages of swallowing.

2. To tolerate the transnasal tube placement, local anesthesia is required.

3. It is invasive and may interfere with swallowing in some patients (Logemann, 1998). Although not documented, difficulty with nasal obstruction

by the tube in bottle-fed infants with respiratory compromise is intuitively suspected.

4. It does not comprehensively assess swallowing physiology.

5. Although there are clinical reports that FEES is commonly used to assess swallowing function in young children (Willging, 1995), other reports indicate that children under 6 to 8 years of age do not tolerate the FEES procedures (Logemann, 1998).

Videofluoroscopic Swallow Study

Videofluoroscopic swallow study (VFSS) is also referred to as oropharyngeal motility study (OPM). Procedures for conducting a VFSS are described in detail later in this section. In general, a VFSS is a radiographic procedure in which all stages of swallowing are video tape recorded in real time and can be analyzed frame by frame. Depending on the equipment used, the video images can be "captured" on a computer, and still x-ray films can be made. The infant is fed formula and/or food mixed with liquid barium, paste barium, or barium powder. Other radio-opaque materials can be used to mix with the food if a fistula is suspected

ADVANTAGES

1. VFSS assesses all stages of the physiology of deglutition in real time.

2. It provides information on bolus transit times, motility disorders, and amount and cause of aspiration.

3. Any video tape recorder can be attached to the fluoroscopic equipment.

4. Strategies to improve swallowing function are assessed during the study, and the effects of these therapeutic interventions on swallowing integrity are known immediately.

5. The video tape recordings can be used for patient/family education and shared with other professionals as part of a multidisciplinary treatment approach.

DISADVANTAGES

1. Although the patient is exposed to small amounts of radiation, this can be a source of concern if the patient requires frequent reassessments.

2. The equipment is not portable; medically fragile children must be transported to the radiology department.

3. The radiographic image that is projected requires training and expertise to correctly delineate anatomic structures and abnormalities.

4. Sensory deficits may be inferred based on a patient's performance; however, no direct sensory testing is conducted.

Cervical Auscultation

Cervical auscultation (CA) is a method of augmenting clinical feeding evaluation by using a stethoscope held against the neck above the larynx to listen to the sounds of swallowing and respiration. CA is not a new technique and has been used with young infants to describe bolus transit through the pharynx, swallow breath sounds, laryngeal and/or nasal penetration of liquid, laryngeal stridor, and changes in respiration/vocalization as a result of pharyngeal dysphagia (Vice, Heinz, Giuriati, Hood, & Bosma, 1990). The sounds of pharyngeal dysphagia in infants during bottle feeding detected using CA include bubbling sounds corresponding to respiration, coughing, clearing, or stridor (Vice, Bamford, Heinz, & Bosma, 1994). CA can be used to identify respiratory status before the introduction of food, during the swallow, and after the swallow to assess the quality of respiration after the ingestion of food.

ADVANTAGES

1. CA is a noninvasive observational procedure used to augment clinical assessment.

2. It can be used to augment a clinical evaluation.

3. It provides a continuous way of monitoring swallowing behaviors.

4. It is inexpensive and portable.

DISADVANTAGES

1. CA is an observational measure that may not be a valid indicator of aspiration when used alone.

2. The sounds of swallowing may be distorted depending on the type of stethoscope used (Hamlet, Penny, & Formolo, 1994).

Evaluation of Feeding/Swallowing

Evaluation of pediatric dysphagia may be accomplished through indepth clinical assessment of feeding and videofluoroscopic swallow study (VFSS). Ideally, a child should receive the clinical assessment first, followed by the VFSS if indicated. The general purposes of these diagnostic methods include:

Clinical Assessment

- Analyze typical feeding behavior
- Obtain social, medical, developmental, and feeding histories
- Examine anatomic structure and function of the oral cavity (jaw, tongue, lips)
- Determine if the infant needs a VFSS
- Determine if the infant can tolerate VFSS procedures
- Assess cranial nerve function for swallowing
- Determine factors affecting normal development of feeding skills

VFSS

- Examine anatomic structure and function of oral, nasal, and pharyngeal cavities simultaneously
- Assess the oral, pharyngeal, and esophageal stages of swallowing and their interaction
- Objectively measure coordination of suck-swallow-breathe sequence
- Determine the maintenance of airway protection during swallowing
- Determine the presence of premature spillage, laryngeal penetration, aspiration and/or residue

- Determine whether the child is at risk for aspiration

- Assess the reactions to swallowing dysfunction and/or aspiration, including protective or clearing reactions
- Assess the response to therapeutic interventions/compensatory strategies
- Make safe feeding recommendations
- Improve feeding efficiency

Signs or symptoms indicating the need for a clinical assessment of feeding/swallowing are listed below. These symptoms may be indicative of serious medical conditions as well as feeding/swallowing problems and therefore may warrant other medical testing.

❖ FTT or sudden weight loss

❖ Sudden change in feeding

❖ Behavioral changes (e.g., fussiness) during or after feeding

❖ Frequent and copious "spitting up"

❖ Bottle feeding lasts more than 30 minutes

❖ Behavioral feeding problems (food refusal, texture aversion)

❖ Weak dysfunctional suck and/or suspected neurologic problems

❖ Coughing/choking during feeding

❖ Change in physiological state during/after feeding

It is important to note that not all infants with dysphagia require a VFSS. A VFSS recommendation should be made only if:

❖ Clinical signs of swallowing dysfunction were noted that warrant an objective evaluation.

❖ The child has a history of repeated upper respiratory infections and/or unexplained pneumonia.

❖ Emesis or other symptoms of GER are present. (Although the VFSS is not the test of choice to study GER, it can provide information regarding structural integrity and possible aspiration after GER episodes.)

❖ The child's medical condition is stable enough so that PO feedings may begin after the VFSS if indicated.

❖ The child is at least 38 weeks of age.

CLINICAL FEEDING EVALUATION OF INFANTS AND OLDER CHILDREN

The following information on clinical assessment was compiled from Alexander, Boehme, and Cupps (1993), Cherney (1994), and Jelm (1990). The clinical assessment can be divided into six parts:

History

Behavior/State/Sensory Integration

General Postural Control/Tone

Respiratory Function/Endurance

Oral-Motor/Cranial Nerve Evaluation

Feeding/Swallowing Evaluation

Information on how to perform a clinical assessment is presented in Forms 3–1 and 3–2 on pages 100 and 106, respectively. Form 3–1 outlines the pertinent medical and social history information that may be obtained as a questionnaire for the parent/caregiver or by a thorough chart review. Form 3–2 walks you through a clinical evaluation of pediatric dysphagia. Table 3–1 shows how to convert ounces and pounds to grams when calculating weight.

The following text briefly describes the information obtained in each section of a clinical assessment.

History

The most important part of the feeding/swallowing evaluation is an indepth case history. By completing Form 3–1, you should know:

1. **Current Status**
   - ❖ medical diagnosis, present concerns, and a brief description of the reason for the referral
   - ❖ birth weight, current weight, gestational age, date of birth, and post-conceptional age

2. **Social History**
   - ❖ family, parent/caregiver relationship, siblings, home environment, and feeding environment

3. **Medical History**
   - ❖ neonatal/birth history, pregnancy history, and delivery history
   - ❖ Apgar scores
   - ❖ perinatal complications
   - ❖ current diagnosis
   - ❖ anesthesia during birth
   - ❖ respiratory history, ventilatory support
   - ❖ current medications
   - ❖ past surgeries
   - ❖ genetic/neurologic testing

TABLE 3–1. Conversion of Pounds and Ounces to Grams When Calculating Infant Weight (Example: To obtain grams equivalent to 2 pounds 8 ounces, read "2" on the top scale, "8" on the side scale; equivalent is 1134 grams.)

	0	1	2	3	4	5	6	7	8	9	10	11	12	13	14
0	0	454	907	1361	1814	2268	2722	3175	3629	4082	4536	4990	5443	5897	6350
1	28	482	936	1389	1843	2296	2750	3203	3657	4111	4564	5018	5471	5925	6379
2	57	510	964	1417	1871	2325	2778	3232	3685	4139	4593	5046	5500	5953	6407
3	85	539	992	1446	1899	2353	2807	3260	3714	4167	4621	5075	5528	5982	6435
4	113	567	1021	1474	1928	2381	2835	3289	3742	4196	4649	5103	5557	6010	6464
5	142	595	1049	1503	1956	2410	2863	3317	3770	4224	4678	5131	5585	6038	6492
6	170	624	1077	1531	1984	2438	2892	3345	3799	4252	4706	5160	5613	6067	6520
7	198	652	1106	1559	2013	2466	2920	3374	3827	4281	4734	5188	5642	6095	6549
8	227	680	1134	1588	2041	2495	2948	3402	3856	4309	4763	5216	5670	6123	6577
9	255	709	1162	1616	2070	2523	2977	3430	3884	4337	4791	5245	5698	6152	6605
10	283	737	1191	1644	2098	2551	3005	3459	3912	4366	4819	5273	5727	6180	6634
11	312	765	1219	1673	2126	2580	3033	3487	3941	4394	4848	5301	5755	6209	6662
12	340	794	1247	1701	2155	2608	3062	3515	3969	4423	4876	5330	5783	6237	6690
13	369	822	1276	1729	2183	2637	3090	3544	3997	4451	4904	5358	5812	6265	6719
14	397	850	1304	1758	2211	2665	3118	3572	4026	4479	4933	5386	5840	6294	6747
15	425	879	1332	1786	2240	2693	3147	3600	4054	4508	4961	5415	5868	6322	6776

Note: 1 pound = 454 grams; 1 ounce = 28 grams; 1000 grams = 1 kilogram.
Gram equivalents have been rounded to whole numbers by adding 1 when the first decimal place is 5 or greater.

❖ relevant lab reports (Hematocrit is the percent of red blood cells in the total blood volume and is normally 50–70% in full-term infants. The reticulocyte count is used to determine bone marrow activity and is normally 4–5% in full-term infants and 6–10 in preterm infants 30–36 weeks gestational age. The reticulocyte count is elevated after a hemorrhage and lower in hemolytic diseases. Bilirubin is the orange-yellow pigment of bile formed by the breakdown of hemoglobin in red blood cells after they naturally die.) *These measures basically tell you if the baby is making enough red blood cells for energy.*

❖ ear infections

❖ sleep patterns

❖ current interventions

❖ allergies

❖ motor development and speech and language information

❖ personality

4. **Feeding and Swallowing History**

❖ feeding development

❖ tube feeding history

❖ weight gain history reflux/emesis during and after meals

❖ aversive behaviors associated with feedings

After collecting the pertinent history information, you are ready to begin your clinical assessment. The following information, presented in Form 3–2, is obtained during a clinical assessment of feeding and swallowing.

Behavior/State/Sensory Integration

1. Note infant's stage of alertness before and after feeding. The goal to is determine the optimal stage(s) of alertness for feeding.

   Stage 1: Deep sleep

   Stage 2: Light sleep

   Stage 3: Drowsy-semidozing

   Stage 4: Quiet alert

   Stage 5: Active alert

   Stage 6: Alert agitated

   Stage 7: Crying

2. Note any stress cues during or after feeding. The goal is to determine the child's tolerance of feeding.

   State-related: staring, looking panicked or hyperalert, silent crying, discharge smiling, dozing, and startle

Motor-related: facial grimmacing; twitching; hyperextension of trunk, arms, hands, or legs

Autonomic (mild): gasp, sigh, sneeze, sweating, hiccup, tremor, startle, and strain

Autonomic (severe): coughing, gag, reflux, skin color change, respiratory pausing, and irregular respiration

3. Note infant's response to touch or stimulation. The goal is to rule out hypersensitivity versus hyposensitivity as factors affecting feeding.

General Postural Control/Tone

Examine general postural control and muscle tone as it affects feeding. Your goals are to achieve the best postural support and muscle tone for successful feeding. For infants, normal posture is a natural, flexed position. The head should be forward in a loose chin tuck position. The shoulders should be symmetrical and slightly depressed. For older children sitting in chairs during feeding, the trunk should be stable and in alignment with the head, neck, and spine. The feet should be supported with the pelvis at a 90° angle. The shoulder girdle should be stable. During this part of the evaluation you will:

❖ assess muscle tone/posture/movement abnormalities

❖ evaluate head/neck/trunk alignment

❖ evaluate the dissassociation of the head/neck from the shoulder girdle (head support)

❖ note abnormal compensatory behaviors

Respiratory Function/Endurance

One of the most common causes of dysphagia in children is related to respiratory problems. If the child is not able to protect the airway during feedings, then the child is not a candidate for oral feedings. Your goal is to observe respiratory patterns both before and after feeding to determine if the child can be fed orally.

❖ respiratory patterns at rest and during activity

❖ respiratory patterns

belly breathing

gulp breathing

ribcage flaring

sternum depression

reverse breathing

irregular/shallow

❖ apnea

Oral-Motor/Cranial Nerve Evaluation

Note oral-motor problems that would interfere with feeding. This important part of the assessment will identify therapy objectives.

Oral Primitive Reflexes

Persistent primitive reflexes may interfere with feeding. This part of the assessment allows you to test for the presence of primitive reflexes that were presented in detail in Table 1–4 (see p. 7).

Oral Structure and Function

The structures and imitative movements that underlie successful feeding are presented. For the infant, much of your evaluation is through observation of the anatomical structures at rest. For the older child who can imitate oral movements, the function can be assessed.

LIPS

- ❖ Observe the lips at rest and note the symmetry of the lip corners.

- ❖ Observe bilabial closure when the child's teeth or gums are together.

- ❖ Ask the child to "Be quiet for a minute." The older child should be able to maintain lip closure for up to 5 seconds.

- ❖ Observe the upper and lower lip separately for increased, decreased, or normal tone.

- ❖ Note anatomical deviancies such as scarring or clefting.

Examine the symmetry and range of motion of upper/lower lip movement by asking the child to imitate the following as you do them:

- ❖ Observe lip opening and closing independent from jaw movement. Say, "Keep your teeth together but open and close your lips like a fish."

- ❖ Observe lip rounding. Say, "Pucker up like you were going to blow a kiss."

- ❖ Observe lip spreading. Say, "Give me your biggest smile."

- ❖ Note the strength of lip resistance. Say, "Keep your lips together and don't let me pull them apart."

- ❖ Note abnormal movement patterns such as lip/cheek retraction (lips/cheeks are pulled backward, with the lips forming a horizontal line) or lip pursing (a movement response to lip/cheek retraction in which the lips pucker but corners remain retracted).

TONGUE

- ❖ Observe tongue size relative to the size of the oral cavity/mandible. Is it too large (macroglossia) or small (microglossia)?

❖ Note any movement abnormalities such as fasciculations and tremors. The tongue should be quiet, at rest on the floor of the mouth.

❖ Note any atrophy by circling R (right), L (left), or G (general).

❖ Note if the tongue is held in a protruded or retracted position at rest.

❖ Look at the contour of the tongue and note if it is flat, thick, or bunched.

❖ Observe the tongue for increased or decreased tone.

❖ Note any lingual deviancies such as scarring or a short lingual frenum. If the frenum is too short, there will be a dimpling of the tongue tip.

Examine the symmetry and range of motion of tongue movements by asking the child to imitate the following as you do them:

❖ Observe protrusion, retraction, and lateralization independent from jaw movement or lip assistance. If necessary, you may have to help the child keep his or her jaw open and stationary when performing the following imitative task. Say, "Open your mouth and stick out your tongue but don't touch your lips. Now pull your tongue back in your mouth. Touch the corners of your lips with the tip of your tongue."

❖ Note degree of tongue tip and back elevation independent of jaw movement or lip assistance. Say, "Open your mouth then try to touch your nose with your tongue. Keep your mouth open and say 'goggle'."

❖ Demonstrate tongue cupping with the lateral edges of your tongue curved upward and the tongue blade held in a bowl shape.

❖ Assess lingual strength by asking the child to press his or her tongue against the inside of the cheek and keep it there while you press against the cheek. Look for weakness to the resistance.

❖ Observe abnormal movement patterns. Strong or forceful protrusion is tongue thrusting. In exaggerated tongue protrusion, the tongue appears thick and moves in a suckling motion.

JAW

❖ Observe the size of the jaw relative to the size of the oral cavity/tongue. Is the jaw too large (macrognathia) or too small (micrognathia)?

❖ Note position of jaw (protruded, retracted, or clenched).

Examine the symmetry and range of motion of jaw movements by asking the child to imitate the following as you do them.

❖ Observe symmetry and degree of jaw opening. Say, "Slowly open your mouth as wide as you can." Note the range of motion and symmetry of jaw excursion.

❖ Ask the child to "Stick out your jaw and move it from side-to-side. Now move it in and out."

❖ Assess strength by asking the child to "Keep your mouth closed; don't let me open it." Attempt to open the mouth by pulling down on the child's chin with your thumb. You can also try "Open your mouth, don't let me close it." Attempt to close the mouth by pushing up on the child's chin with your thumb.

❖ Observe abnormal movements such as jaw thrusting, where the jaw moves downward in a strong, forceful manner.

Examine the dental bite and note any maloccusions.

MALOCCLUSIONS

1. **Neutrocclusion:** Angle's Class I. Molars are in proper alignment but there are other dental problems such as missing teeth or tooth positions.

2. **Distocclusion:** Angle's Class II. Mandibular molars are too far posterior in relation to the maxillary molars, giving the look of a retruded mandible.

3. **Mesiocclusion:** Angle's Class III. Mandibular molars are too far anterior in relation to the maxillary molars, giving the look of a protruded mandible.

DENTAL BITE

1. **Openbite:** The upper and lower incisors, and possible canines, do not meet.

2. **Overbite:** The upper incisors overlap the lower incisors with a significant gap between them.

3. **Overjet:** The upper incisors project in front of the lower incisors creating a space.

4. **Underjet:** The upper incisors project behind the lower incisors creating a space.

5. **Crossbite:** Maxillary and mandibular teeth are not vertically aligned. In some cases, for example, the right lower canine may be in contact with the upper left incisor.

Cranial Nerve Screening

A full assessment of cranial nerve function is presented in Table 3–2. A cranial nerve screening of CN V, VII, X and XII is included within Form 3–2 (see p. 108).

Feeding/Swallowing Evaluation

During a clinical examination, you can assess the oral preparatory/oral stage of swallowing as well as make inferences regarding the pharyngeal stage. The goal is to identify oral preparatory/oral stage problems and solutions to address them. If you suspect pharyngeal stage problems after this feeding evaluation, the child may need a VFSS.

Bottle Feeding

❖ evaluate NS versus NNS (see Form 3–3 on p. 113)

❖ note type of bottle, type of liquid, flow of nipple

TABLE 3–2. Assessment of Cranial Nerves in Feeding/Swallowing

CRANIAL NERVE V (TRIGEMINAL-Mandibular Branch)

Innervation: muscles of mastication (masseter), soft palate (tensor veli palatini), mylohyoid, anterior belly of digastric

- **Motor:** mastication (jaw closing and lateral jaw movement) in the Oral Stage; assists in upward/anterior movement of the larynx; backward movement of the tongue to the soft palate, movement of the tensor veli palatini, palatal elevation and posterior pharyngeal wall constriction (Pharyngeal Stage), lowering of the palate after the swallow
- **Sensory:** sensation to the superficial and deep structures of the face, mucous membrane of the upper mouth, palate, tongue; sensation of shape and texture in the mouth (Oral Stage), sensation to the palate and pharynx (Pharyngeal Stage)

Assessment

1. Observe face at rest and look for unilateral or bilateral drooping or clenching.
2. Observe contours of the temporalis and masseter muscles at rest.
3. "Bite down and show me your teeth." Palpate masseter and feel for unilateral or bilateral weakness.
4. "Keep you mouth closed. Don't let me open it." Attempt to open the mouth by pulling down on the child's chin with your thumb. Note strength of resistance.
5. "Open your mouth. Don't let me close it." Attempt to close the mouth by pushing up on the child's chin with your thumb. Note the range of motion and symmetry of jaw excursion.
6. "Stick your jaw out and move it side to side." With unilateral paralysis, the jaw will deviate to the paralyzed side.
7. For an older verbal child give the following instruction. "Close your eyes." Then lightly touch one side of the face with the tip of a pencil, then touch the other. Ask the child to describe the sensation; compare the two sides and ask the child to show you the first place that was touched.
8. Ask the child to open and close his/her mouth as fast as she or he can. Look for slow, rapid or irregular movements. Also note any tremors or involuntary movements (fasciculations).

CRANIAL NERVE VII (FACIAL)

Innervation: muscles of facial expression (orbicularis oculi and oris, zygomatic, buccinator, platysma), stylohyoid, posterior belly of digastric

- **Motor:** movements involved with facial expression; assists with elevation of the larynx; lip and face muscles allow food to be held inside the mouth (Oral Phase), movement of the palate, elevation of the hyoid and tongue (Pharyngeal Stage). Facial muscles below the forehead receive contralateral innervation. The frontalis muscle (forehead) receives bilateral innervation.
- **Sensory:** taste to the anterior two thirds of the tongue; sensation to the floor of the mouth, hard palate and soft palate; taste sensation to the tongue (Oral Stage)

Assessment

1. Observe the face at rest and during facial expressions. Look for "masked" or limited facial expressions and symmetry of movement.
2. Observe the corners of the mouth. Asymmetric drooping may indicate unilateral damage to CN VII.
3. "Look straight at me. Now, don't move your head and look way up at the ceiling." Or "Wrinkle your forehead." Weakness or inability to wrinkle the forehead may indicate peripheral damage to CN VII or contralateral cortical damage.
4. "Close your eyes and don't let me open them." Note strength of resistance.
5. "Smile" or "Close your eyes as tightly as you can." Note symmetry of retraction of the corners of the mouth.
6. "Puff up your cheeks with air and don't let me squeeze it out." Gently squeeze the cheeks together and note strength of resistance.
7. "Show me a pouting face" or "Pull down the corners of your mouth." Look for weakness, tremors, or any involuntary movements.
8. Take three cups and place water in the first, a 50/50 water/lemon juice solution in the second, and straight lemon juice in the third. Instruct the child "Tell me what this tastes like." Using a cotton swab, start with the water and place a drop of each solution on the child's tongue. Note child's reaction to taste.

CRANIAL NERVE IX (GLOSSOPHARYNGEAL)

Innervation: stylopharyngeal muscle, pharynx (portion of the middle pharyngeal constrictor), parotid salivary gland

- **Motor:** elevation of the larynx and pharynx through the sylopharyngeus muscle; palatal movement, pharyngeal and laryngeal movement, epiglottic excursion (Pharyngeal Stage)

- **Sensory:** taste and general sensation to the posterior one third of the tongue, sensation to tonsils, upper pharynx, and soft palate; glossopharyngeal portion mediates the sensory portion of the pharyngeal gag; taste to the tongue (Oral Phase), sensation to the palate and tongue (Pharyngeal Stage)

Assessment

1. Observe the velum at rest and then ask the child to say "Ah, Ah, Ah" forcefully. Note unilateral or bilateral drooping (CN IX and X). The uvula will point toward the nondamaged side (away from the weak side).
2. Test for the strength of the gag reflex (CN IX and X). Look for hyper- and hyposensitivity, unilateral loss of the gag reflex.
3. "Close your eyes and stick out your tongue. Tell me which one feels big and soft and which one feels small and hard." Use the wood-tipped end of a sterile cotton swab and then the cotton swab end to touch the tip of the tongue.

CRANIAL NERVE X (VAGUS)

Innervation: muscles of the soft palate (except tensor veli palitini), pharynx (inferior, middle, and superior pharyngeal constrictors), intrinsic muscles of the larynx (cricothyroid, thyroarytenoid, posterior cricoarytenoid, lateral cricoarytenoid, interarytenoids), various muscles of the esophagus

- **Motor:** elevation and depression of the soft palate, elevation and closure of the larynx, movement of the pharynx and esophagus; epiglottic excursion, opening of the cricopharyngeal segment (Pharyngeal Stage), esophageal peristalsis, lowering of the larynx after the swallow
- **Sensory:** sensation to the pharynx, larynx, trachea, lungs, epiglottis; movement of the palate, laryngeal elevation, pharyngeal contraction, sensation to the larynx and pharynx, epiglottis

Assessment

1. Listen for the voice quality (gurgly or "wet," breathiness, hoarseness, stridor, diplophonia, tremors, resonance problems, etc.).
2. Test for strength of glottic closure. "Cough hard." Experience suggests that you instruct the child to cover his/her mouth before executing this command.
3. Observe the velum (see above).
4. Ask the child to swallow. Evidence of CN X damage will become apparent during the clinical feeding/swallowing evaluation (i.e., reduced laryngeal closure, delay in swallow response).

CRANIAL NERVE XII (HYPOGLOSSAL)

Innervation: intrinsic muscles of the tongue and some of the extrinsic muscles of the tongue: superior longitudinal, inferior longitudinal, transverse, verticalis, genioglossus, hyoglossus, and styloglossus

- **Motor:** controls tongue movement (intrinsic muscles control tongue shortening, concaving [cupping], narrowing, elongating, and flattening; extrinsic muscles are responsible for drawing the tongue upward, forward and backward, retraction and depression); movements of the tongue, backward movement of the tongue to the soft palate (Oral Stage), elevation of the hyoid bone and tongue (Pharyngeal Stage)
- **Sensory:** none

Assessment

1. Observe the tongue at rest. Note fasciculations, tremors, and atrophy.
2. "Stick out your tongue." Observe independent tongue movement without jaw assistance. Also note symmetry of protrusion. The tongue will deviate toward the side of lesion (away from the strong side).
3. "Stick out your tongue and don't let me push it back in your mouth." Encourage the child not to use his/her lips to hold the tongue out.
4. "Stick out your tongue and don't let me push it over." Check lateral resistance to tongue blade by placing the blade on one side of the tongue and trying to push the tongue over to the other side. You can also ask the child to press his or her tongue against the inside of the cheek and keep it there while you press against the cheek. Look for weakness.
5. "Move your tongue from side to side." Encourage the child not to use his or her jaw to move the tongue.
6. "Open your mouth as wide as you can and then touch your tongue to the roof of your mouth." Look for range of motion, ability to lift tongue from floor of mouth. Depending on how widely the child opens his or her mouth, she or he normally may not be able to make contact with the palate.

Sources: Compiled from Love, R. J. & Webb, W. G. (1996). *Neurology for the speech-language pathologist* (3rd ed.). Newton: Butterworth-Heinemann; Wolf, L. S., & Glass, R. P. (1992). *Feeding and swallowing disorders in infancy.* Tuscon: Therapy Skill Builders. Perlman, X., Perlman, A., & Schulze-Delrieu, X. (1997). *Deglutition and its disorders: Anatomy, physiology, clinical diagnosis and management.* San Diego: Singular Publishing Group. Perlman, A. (2000, February). *Clinical evaluation of feeding and swallowing in school aged children.* Paper presented at the 40th annual Illinois Speech Hearing Association. Arlington Park, IL.

- ❖ note position
- ❖ suckle initiation (suckle lag?)
- ❖ strength of tongue seal (0–6 months)
- ❖ strength of lip seal (6 months and up)
- ❖ suckle versus sucking
- ❖ mandibular excursion
- ❖ cervical auscultation
- ❖ suck(le)/swallow ratio at beginning versus end of feeding
- ❖ length of burst cycle
- ❖ length of feeding (endurance)

Cup Drinking

- ❖ lip/cheek movements
- ❖ tongue movements
- ❖ jaw stability
- ❖ biting cup
- ❖ loss of material

Straw Drinking

- ❖ lip/tongue/cheek movements
- ❖ vary viscosity of liquids; can they control volume?

Spoon Feeding

- ❖ anticipatory open mouth
- ❖ jaw gradation
- ❖ lip/tongue/cheek movement
- ❖ clean spoon? How?

Biting/Chewing Soft Solid

- ❖ anterior munching pattern (early)
  - • straight movement of jaw up/down
  - • diagonal munch pattern: food moves side to side
- ❖ mature rotary chewing pattern (later)
  - • bite/grind
- ❖ open mouth or lip closure?
- ❖ lip/tongue/cheek/jaw movements.

Biting/Chewing Hard Solid

- ❖ tongue lateralization
  - midline to side
  - side, midline to side
  - side to side

Cervical Auscultation

Cervical auscultation can be used to augment a traditional feeding evaluation. A pediatric stethoscope is placed near the larynx and the sounds of swallowing/respiration are observed.

- ❖ Start by listening to normal respiration before introducing food.
- ❖ Listen to the cycles of sucking/swallowing/breathing.
- ❖ Listen for the timing of the swallow response.
- ❖ Observe change in respiratory sound after the swallow (be careful only to document that respiratory sounds did or did not change).

VIDEOFLUOROSCOPIC SWALLOW STUDY

The VFSS is a collaborative effort between the radiologist and the feeding specialist (i.e., speech-language pathologist). Before scheduling the VFSS, the feeding specialist should brief the radiologist regarding the results of the clinical assessment, other pertinent medical information, and objectives for the study. The feeding specialist is responsible for (a) positioning the infant/child, (b) assembling the feeding equipment, (c) instructing the parent/caretaker who acts as the feeder during the study, (d) assuming the role of feeder if necessary, (e) working with the radiologist to obtain the optimum view, (f) helping the infant/child to maintain midline head positioning, (g) evaluating the stages of swallowing, and (h) making suggestions for intervention and/or compensatory strategies. The radiologist is responsible for (a) reviewing prior films, (b) diagnosing anatomical abnormalities, (c) assessing the adequacy of airway protection and swallowing parameters in conjunction with the feeding specialist, (d) screening the esophageal stage, and (e) reviewing the videotape with the feeding specialist to discuss objective findings.

Because the VFSS involves radiation exposure, the time in which the infant/child is exposed should be kept to a minimum. The limitations are usually set by the radiology department and typically run between 2–5 minutes.

Conducting and Evaluating a VFSS

Form 3–4 (see p. 114) outlines the steps in conducting and evaluating a VFSS. The following are some tips to make the VFSS successful.

Getting Started

- ❖ Be sure the child is hungry.
- ❖ Make feeding as familiar/natural as possible (i.e., familiar utensils).

❖ The parent/primary caregiver should feed the child.

❖ Use simultaneous audio and video recordings to document textures/flow rates and so forth given during evaluation.

❖ Use universal precautions (i.e., gloves, shields, glasses, or goggles)

POSITIONING

To achieve optimum views, special seating and positioning devices may be needed. Table 3–3 describes some common pediatric chairs and positioning devices.

❖ For premature or small infants, use a small seat (i.e., Tumbleform™, with appropriate support for the head/neck/trunk at a 45° angle).

❖ For full-term infants and children, use larger seats or special seats (i.e., MAMA™ chair).

VIEW

❖ Start with a lateral view with the field open to the lips, velopharyngeal port, and upper one third of the esophagus. Only do an A/V view if aspiration occurs. Keep the study under 2 minutes. Be sure to use fluoroscopy to examine the beginning, middle, and end of feedings.

TABLE 3–3. Pediatric Videofluoroscopic Swallow Studies Evaluation Chairs

During a pediatric videofluoroscopic swallow study, we are trying to simulate how the child eats at home and also determine ways to promote successful feeding. It would be ideal to use the child's own seating system. Most facilities do not utilize portable C-arms and, unfortunately, most chairs (high chairs, wheelchairs, and car seats) do not fit between the fluoroscopic table and the filming surface. Other problems include metal head rests and seat height, which can obstruct the view.

The following information is a guide for seating/positioning options you may encounter with pediatric patients. Regardless of the systems used, proper trunk alignment as well as head and neck support must be attained.

• The Hausted Video-Fluoroscopic Imaging Chair™ is appropriate for older children. It offers a variety of options, including waist, torso, and leg velcro restraint straps; foot pedal hydraulics for height adjustments; and side rails to help patients with neurological problems maintain their posture. Another feature that increases the chair's safety is its transportability. The chair's backrest can be lowered to allow a patient to be easily transferred from a bed to the chair and then wheeled to the Radiology Department.

• The VESS Chair™ is also designed for older children and adults. It comes with IV stand holder, chart holder, oxygen tank holder, Foley bag holder, removable arms, linear actuator tilting device, and a front wheel-locking mechanism for better steering control. This chair is adaptable to mobility impaired patients, tilts for accommodation of flexed patients, and is easy to transport patient from bed to the Imaging Department. Safety features include a lap belt, plus torso and leg restraining straps. Head control and patient comfort can be enhanced with attachable bean bag pillows and head control strap.

• For young children and infants, depending on the child's size, an insert, such as a small Tumble Form Seat™ with appropriate support for the trunk, neck, and head, may be used in addition to these adult evaluation chairs. Medium and large Tumble Form Seats™ are available for larger children. Additionally, car seats can be adapted to fit in an upright fluoroscopic table.

• Some hospitals may own a chair specific to evaluating the pediatric population. The MAMA™ (Multiple Application Multiple Articulation) is a common chair used during pediatric swallow evaluations. It has a variety of adjustment capabilities useful in getting children with significant physical impairments into an appropriate position for feeding. It can be moved easily so the child can be positioned outside the radiology suite and wheeled into position without taking additional time during the evaluation. It accommodates newborn infants and children up to 5 feet tall.

MATERIALS

❖ Figure 3–1 illustrates a variety of feeding utensils that may be used during a VFSS. You should have several nipples ready (preemie, regular, low flow, Haberman). See Section 7, Resources, "Feeding Equipment and Distributors" on p. 201 for a listing of various nipples/bottles.

❖ Infants who readily, easily, and quickly consume formula or breast milk are labeled "good feeders." One of the first types of therapeutic intervention with "poor feeders" is to increase the flow rate of the liquid from the nipple. Schrank, Al-Sayed, Beahm, and Thach (1998) define slow flow rates as 3.6 ml/minute and high flow rates as 16.2 ml/minute. In general, increasing flow rate results in a higher suck/swallow ratio. Both "healthy" term and preterm infants have been reported to tolerate increases in flow rate (Schrank et al., 1998), but care must be taken to carefully monitor stress cues from the premature infant.

❖ Have glucose, formula, or breast milk that is not mixed with barium ready to continue feedings between fluoroscopic imaging. Have all appropriate consistencies ready and mixed with either liquid, paste, or powder barium. Have parents bring in the food (easiest to hardest consistency). Other utensils possibly needed are:

various cups (cut out, flow-guard lid)

straw

spoons (different sizes and one with a shallow bowl)

syringe

pacifier

different bottles and nipples with low-fast flow rates and various nipple sizes

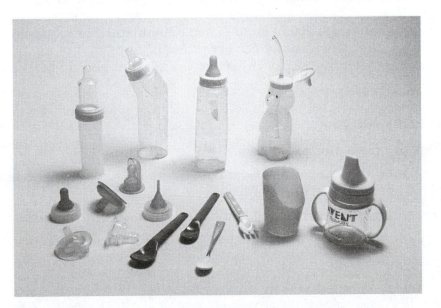

Figure 3–1. Examples of feeding utensils that may be used during a videofluoroscopic swallow study.

Procedures

PRESENTATIONS

❖ For infants receiving primary enteral feedings, begin with establishing an NNS. Next, introduce nipple feedings using a regular or preemie nipple with a regular flow rate. For older children, liquids may be presented via spoon (2 ml). Increase quantity and texture and vary the utensils.

❖ For children currently receiving PO feedings, start with the easiest consistency. First establish a nonnutritive sucking, then introduce familiar bottle feeding to allow comparison of NS and NNS. Do not regulate the feedings. With older children, we typically begin with spoon feedings. Instruct the parent/caregiver to feed the infant as done at home.

Interpretations/Recommendations

Swallowing function can vary depending on the utensil or food used. Here are some important things to remember when evaluating swallowing function using VFSS.

❖ Infants trigger at the vallecula by tongue pressing the posterior pharyngeal wall.

❖ This is a tongue back/down pattern and is different from older children who use a tongue back/up pattern, triggering at the anterior faucial pillars.

❖ Some infants experience vestibular penetration during the initial suckle burst. This penetration, if normal, will clear after the first few swallows (Beecher, 1994).

Stages of Feeding/Swallowing

Logemann (1998) divides the process of deglutition into four stages. In the oral preparatory stage, food is prepared for swallowing. In the oral stage, food is transported posteriorly through the oral cavity. The swallowing response is triggered in the pharyngeal stage. Here, food safely passes around the closed larynx into the esophagus to begin the esophageal stage. Each stage is age dependent. For example, oral preparation to swallow in a newborn would be very different from that of an 18-month-old infant. The following is a summary of the major events that should be evaluated in each stage of swallowing.

Oral Preparatory Stage

1. **Suck(l)ing from the nipple**

   ❖ The infant *latches* onto the nipple when presented to the lips with a tight lip or tongue seal.

   ❖ The infant immediately begins tongue/jaw movements to *initiate sucking.*

   ❖ *Rhythymic sucking* at a rate of 1–2 sucks per swallow/breath

   ❖ *Stripping the nipple*

   ❖ *Nipple compression*

   ❖ *Posterior nipple placement*

2. Removing food from spoon

❖ Mouth opening

❖ Closure around spoon

❖ Lip assistance to remove food

3. *Mastication (or munching)* of soft solids (with or without teeth present) or *mashing* (between gums or tongue and hard palate)

4. *Manipulating* the food from side to side to *form* a bolus

5. Holding the food midline on the dorsum of the tongue in preparation to swallow. Liquids may be held in the mouth up to 2–3 seconds.

6. Utensil use: spoon, fork, cup, and so forth

Oral Stage

1. Posterior transit of the bolus

2. Oral transit time is timed from the first posterior movement until the bolus head reaches the ramus of the mandible (a radiographic landmark) (Logemann, 1998).

3. Lingual peristalsis (toddler/older child)

4. Tongue contact with hard and soft palate

5. Soft palate elevates simultaneously with the triggering of the swallowing response.

Pharyngeal Stage

1. Begins with elicitation of *swallow response* and ends with the bolus passing the CP segment

2. Laryngeal elevation (length of excursion increases with age) and anterior movement

3. *Vestibular entry*: normal for liquids to enter the laryngeal vestibule but clear with the swallow during the first few sucks at the beginning of a sucking burst

4. *Epiglottic excursion*

5. *Pharyngeal contraction*: No *residue*

6. CP dilation

Esophageal Stage

1. *Primary peristalsis*

2. *Secondary peristalsis*

Form 3–1. History Information: Feeding Evaluation Parent/Caregiver Questionnaire

Name of Child _____

Date of birth _____   Chronological Age _____

Gestational Age _____   Current Weight _____

Mother's name and address   Father's name and address

_____   _____

_____   _____

_____   _____

_____   _____

Physician _____   Referred by _____

Reason for Referral _____

Current Status

What is the child's medical diagnosis? _____

What are the present concerns? _____

Has the problem changed? (Gotten better or worse?) _____

Are there any times when the problem is better or worse? _____

_____

Social History

With whom is the child living? _____

Names and ages of siblings _____

Who are the primary caregivers? _____

Who usually feeds the child? _____

Medical History

List maternal illnesses or infections during pregnancy

____Toxemia   ____Bleeding   ____Thyroid disease

Other _____

List any other problems during pregnancy _____

List all medications taken during pregnancy _____

Tests/x-rays during pregnancy _____

Was alcohol or any drug used before/during pregnancy by either parents? _____

Length of pregnancy in weeks _____

Duration of labor _____

Type of delivery _____ Head first _____ Feet first _____ Cesarean _____ Breech

List any problems during labor and delivery _____

Was anesthesia used during birth? (If yes, for what reason?) _____

_____

Apgar Scores _____

Did the child need ventilatory support at birth? _____ Yes _____ No

List any medications that the child is currently taking _____

List and describe any surgeries the child has had _____

Has the child experienced any of the following illnesses?

_____ Ear infections _____ Allergies or asthma _____ High fevers _____ Seizures

_____Frequent upper respiratory infections _____Pneumonia

Other Illnesses: _____

Has any genetic or neurologic testing been conducted? (If yes, explain.) _____

_____

Describe the child's sleep patterns _____

Is the child irritable at times? (if so, when?) _____

Does the child experience frequent constipation? _____

Is the child toilet trained? (circle one)   Bladder: Yes or No

                                                 Bowel: Yes or No

Motor Development

Age the child sat alone _____ Crawled _____

Walked independently _____

Hand preference _____

Describe gross or fine motor problems _____

continued

Communication /Speech and Language history

Quiet, noisy, or average child? _____

At what age did he/she start babbling or imitating sounds? _____

What were the first 3 or 4 words? _____

Age of first word _____

Two-word combinations? When? _____

Estimated number of words in the child's speaking vocabulary _____

Is the child easy or difficult to understand? _____

How does the child communicate needs? _____

What types of questions does the child readily understand? _____

What types of directions are difficult for the child? _____

Describe the child's voice quality:

_____ Breathy _____ Shrill _____ Hypernasal _____ Gurgly _____ Weak _____ Hyponasal

Pitch: _____ normal _____ too high _____ too low

Volume: _____ normal _____ weak _____ loud

Describe the Child's Personality

What are his/her likes and dislikes? _____

What toys and activities does the child enjoy? _____

Any fears? _____

What kinds of situations frustrate the child? _____

For what is the child disciplined? _____

What types of discipline are used? _____

What kinds of things can the child do himself/herself?

_____ Dressing _____ Bathing _____ Toileting _____ Eating

Other _____

What is the child's usual bedtime and rising time? _____

Does the child nap? _____ How long? _____

Are there any sleep problems? _____ Lengthy night wakings _____ Snoring _____ Mouth Breathing

Other: _____

Feeding and Swallowing History

Was the child breast fed?   _____ Yes   _____ No

    For how long? _____

    Were there ever any problems? _____

Was or is the child fed through a feeding tube?   _____ Yes   _____ No

    For how long? _____

What does the child eat in a typical day? List main foods and approximate amounts:

Morning _____

Afternoon _____

Evening _____

Duration of average feeding: How long does it take the child to complete a meal?

____ Less than 10 minutes   ____ 10–20 minutes   ____ 20–30 minutes

____ Over 30 minutes

How many times a day does the child eat? _____

    Estimated amount of liquid consumed per day _____

    Estimated amount of food consumed per day _____

What are the child's favorite foods? _____

What foods/liquids appear to be more difficult for the child to eat? _____

_____

How is the child usually positioned during feeding?

_____ Held on the lap   _____ Infant seat   _____ High chair

_____ Booster seat   _____ Sitting in a chair at the table   _____ Other

_____ Sitting in a wheelchair   _____ Lying down

What utensils are usually used and at what age were they introduced?

Bottle _____   Spoon or fork _____

Fingers _____   Tippy cup _____

Straw _____   Cup (no lid) _____

Other _____

continued

Is adaptive equipment used during feedings?

_____

At what age did the child stop using a bottle? _____

Does the child feed himself/herself?   _____ Yes   _____ No   If yes, with

_____ Fingers   _____ Spoon or fork   _____ Cup/glass   _____ Straw

At what age did the child start feeding himself/herself? _____

What kinds of food does the child eat most of the time?

____ Breast milk   ____ Formula

____ Strained child food   ____ Mashed table food

____ Junior child food   ____ Chopped table food

____ Regular table food   ____ Other

At what age was solid food introduced? _____

What foods does the child **not** like to eat?_____

Does the child take any nutritional supplements? (Product, amount, frequency)

_____

How do you know when the child is hungry? _____

How do you know when the child is full? _____

Please check those that apply to the child:

____Choking during a meal   ____Gagging during a meal

____Food or liquid coming out of nose   ____Cries during meals

____Eats too much   ____Eats too little

____Difficulty swallowing   ____Reflux during/after meals

____Trouble breathing during feeding   ____Emesis during/after meals

____Fussing during feeding   ____Falling asleep during feeding

____Spitting food out   ____Refuses oral feeding

____Postural changes during feeding: ____stiffening   ____hyperextending

____Noisy breathing : During, before, or after feeding?_____

____Gurgly voice quality: During, before, or after feeding?_____

Has the child ever turned blue during or after a feeding? _____

_____

Is the child having trouble gaining weight?   _____ Yes   _____ No

Are mealtimes pleasant?   _____ Yes   _____ No

Does the child have behavior problems during mealtime?   _____ Yes   _____ No

____ Throws food   ____ Messy eater

____ Spits food   ____ Refuses to eat

____ Cries, screams   ____ Takes food from other's plate

____ Leaves table before finished

Does the child use a pacifier?   _____ Yes   _____ No

Does the child have difficulty with the movements of his/her mouth for feeding and/or speech?

_____ Yes   _____ No

Does the child dislike being touched around or in the mouth?   _____ Yes   _____ No

How much does the child drool?

____ Never   ____ Occasionally   ____ Constantly

____ Rarely   ____ Frequently

What seems to help (or not help) the child during mealtime? _____

_____

Form 3–2. Clinical Evaluation of Pediatric Dysphagia

Name: _____ **MR#:** _____ **DOB:** _____

Gestational Age: _____ **Adjusted Age:** _____

Weight at Birth: _____ **Current Weight:** _____

Neonatologist/Physician: _____ **Dx:** _____

Lab Results: _____

DOE: _____ **Examiner:** _____

Behavior/State/Sensory Integration

Physiologic Status

	Before Feedings	**After Feedings**
RR:		
HR:		
SaO^2:		

Stages of Alertness: (BF: before feeding; AF: after feeding)

	Stage 1 Deep Sleep
	Stage 2 Light Sleep
	Stage 3 Dozing/Drowsy
	Stage 4 Quiet Alert
	Stage 5 Active Alert
	Stage 6 Alert Agitated
	Stage 7 Crying

Color: (Before and After)

_____ normal   _____ peri-oral or peri-orbital duskiness   _____ mottled

_____ cyanotic   _____ grey   _____ flushed

_____ ruddy   _____ paling around nostrils

Stress Cues During Feeding

State Related (check)

	Staring
	Panicked, worried, or dull look
	Silent/weak cry
	Discharge smiling
	Dozing
	Startle
	Eye-floating
	Gaze aversion
	Glassy-eyed

Motor Related

	Facial grimacing
	Twitching
	Hyperextension of trunk, arms, hands, or legs
	Fluctuating tone from normal to flaccid
	Hypertonicity (arching, finger splays, fisting)
	Excessive diffuse movements

Autonomic (mild)

	Gasp
	Sigh
	Sneeze
	Sweating
	Hiccup
	Tremor

Autonomic (severe)

	Coughing
	Gagging
	Reflux
	Skin color change
	Respiratory pausing
	Irregular respiration

Infant's response to touch or stimulation: ____ normal   ____ hyposensitive   ____ hypersensitive

General Postural Control/Tone

Overall Muscle tone: ____ Normal   ____ Hypotonic   ____ Hypertonic   ____ Fluctuating

Head/neck/trunk alignment: ____ yes ____ no   Describe: _____

Independent head support: ____ yes ____ no   Describe: _____

Pelvic stability: ____ yes ____ no   Describe: _____

Trunk stability   ____ yes ____ no   Describe: _____

Movements against gravity: ____ yes ____ no   Describe: _____

Problems: ____ hyperextension of the neck (head back) ____ scapula adduction ____ shoulder elevation

____ shoulder retraction

continued

Respiratory/Status   ____ Within normal limits   ____ Breaths per minute

____ Labored/noisy   ____ Mouth breather

____ Stridor   ____ Apnea: describe _____

Abnormal Respiratory Patterns (check pattern)

____ rib cage flaring

____ sternum depression

____ reverse breathing

____ abdominal (belly breathing)

____ irregular/shallow

History of Aspiration _____

Tracheotomy   ____ yes   ____ no   Type _____   Size _____

Position of cuff   ____ Inflated   ____ Partially Inflated   ____ Deflated

Suctioning required   ____ yes   ____ no   Frequency _____

Oral/Motor/Cranial Nerve Evaluation

Oral Primitive Reflexes: (+ = appropriately present − = inappropriately present 0 = absent)

Score	Reflex	Stimulus	Diminishes by
	gag	touch back of tongue	continues through adulthood
	phasic bite	stimulate gums	9–12 months
	transverse tongue	stroke sides of tongue	6 months
	tongue protrusion	touch tongue tip	6 months
	rooting	stroke cheek or corner of mouth	3 months
	sucking/suckling	place nipple in mouth, stroke tongue or touch hard palate	6–24 months

Oral Structure and Function

Lips/Cheeks:

At rest

Lips are symmetrical	___yes	___no (___left ___right)	
Lips touch when teeth are together	___yes	___no	
Lip closure maintained	___yes	___no	
Upper lip tone	___increased	___decreased	___normal
Lower lip tone	___increased	___decreased	___normal
Deviancies	___scar	___ cleft	___other

Imitation

Mvts are symmetrical L/R	___yes	___no (___left ___right)	
Mvts are symmetrical Upper/Lower	___yes	___no (___lupper ___lower)	
Open/close	___normal	___reduced	
Rounding	___normal	___reduced	
Spreading	___normal	___reduced	

Resistance	___normal	___reduced
Problems	___ lip/cheek retraction	__ lip pursing
	___limited upper lip movements	

Tongue

At rest

Size	___large	___small	___normal
Fasciculations/tremors	___yes	___no	
Atrophy	___yes (R/L/G)	___no	
Protruded	___yes	___no	
Retracted	___yes	___no	
Flat	___yes	___no	
Thick	___yes	___no	
Bunched	___yes	___no	
Tone	___increased	___decreased	___normal
Deviancies	___scar	___short frenum	___other

Imitation

Protrusion	___normal	___reduced
Retraction	___normal	___reduced
Lateralization	___normal	___reduced (___left ___right)
Tip elevation	___normal	___reduced
Back elevation	___normal	___reduced
Cupping	___yes	___no
Resistance	___normal	___reduced
Abnormal patterns	___thrusting	___exaggerated protrusion
	___limited movements	

Jaw

At rest

Size	___large	___small	___normal
Protruded	___yes	___no	
Retracted	___yes	___no	
Clenched (tonic bite reflex)	___yes	___no	

Imitation

Graded opening	___normal	___reduced(___left ___right)
Lateralization	___normal	___reduced (___left ___right)
Protrusion	___normal	___reduced
Resistance	___normal	___reduced
Abnormal Patterns	___thrusting	

Malocclusions: _____Neutrocclusion _____Distocclusion

_____Mesiocclusion

Dental Bite: _____Openbite

_____Overjet

_____Underjet

_____Crossbite

continued

Cranial Nerve Screening (note possible CN involvement)

Symptoms

_____ CN V (trigeminal)   reduced mandibular movements

_____ CN VII (facial)   facial asymmetry, reduced facial movements, weak lip closure

_____ CN X (vagus)   vocal fold paralysis, weak cry, hypernasality, nasal regurgitation

_____ CN XII   reduced tongue movements, poor suck

Feeding/Swallowing Evaluation

Nonnutritive Sucking:

     Burst cycles_____

     Endurance: _____ (note when fatigue occurs)

     Lip closure on finger/nipple _____adequate _____weak

     Tongue cupping _____yes _____no

     Strength of suck _____ adequate _____weak

Nutritive Sucking:

     Average length of burst cycles_____

     Length of feeding/Endurance: _____ (note when fatigue occurs)

     Lip/tongue seal on nipple _____adequate _____weak

     Tongue cupping _____yes _____no

     Strength of suck _____ adequate _____weak

     Suckle initiation _____ within normal limits _____ delayed (suckle lag)

Suck(le)/swallow ratio at beginning of feeding:_____

Suck(le)/swallow ratio at end of feeding:_____

Positioning

     Habitual_____

     Trial/Optimal Feeding Position_____

     Assistive Devices (chairs, etc.) _____

Presentation Information

Breast/bottle	**Cup**	**Spoon**	**Bite/chew Soft solids**	**Bite/chew Hard solids**
Bottle type:	Cup type:	Spoon type:	Food type:	Food type:
Liquid type:	Straw:	Liquid type:	chopped/soft_____	chopped/chewey____
thin_____	Liquid type:	thin_____	regular soft_____	regular hard_____
thick_____	thin_____	thick_____		
Nipple flow:		Food type:		
Feeding time:	thick_____	pureed_____		
Position of feeding:		ground_____		
		chopped_____		

Oral-Motor/Swallowing Patterns

KEY: br = breast   bt = bottle   st = straw   c = cup   sp = spoon   ss = soft solids   hs = hard solids

	Lip/Cheek Movement	Tongue Movement	Jaw Movement	Swallowing and Cervical Auscultation
Liquids	____ maintains closure ____ poor lip seal ____ bite/chew ____ active pull on nipple ____ retracted ____ pursed ____ loss of liquid unilateral____ bilateral ____ ____ increased drooling	____ posterior hold ____ anterior hold ____ suckle lag ____ reduced mobility ____ reduced cupping ____ reduced stripping ____ inadequate suck/draw ____ residue ____ pooling ____ tongue thrust ____ retraction ____ cleans lips ____ prolonged oral transit time ____ reduced bolus formation	____ reduced mandibular excursion ____ jaw thrust ____ tonic bite reflex ____ clenching ____ bruxism ____ reduced jaw gradation ____ no anticipatory open mouth ____ biting cup ____ reduced bite/chew	____ delayed trigger pharyngeal swallow ____ absent trigger pharyngeal swallow ____ swallows per bolus ____ wet vocal quality before swallow ____ wet vocal quality after the swallow ____ cough before swallow ____ cough during swallow ____ cough after swallow
	Comments:			

continued

Oral-Motor/Swallowing Patterns

KEY: br = breast   bt = bottle   st = straw   c = cup   sp = spoon   ss = soft solids   hs = hard solids

	Lip/Cheek Movement	Tongue Movement	Jaw Movement	Swallowing and Cervical Auscultation
Solids	____ reduced approximation ____ no active closure ____ no active movement ____ does not maintain closure ____ food loss ____ retracted ____ pursed	____ reduced cupping ____ protrusion ____ reduced bolus formation ____ residue ____ pooling ____ tongue thrust ____ retraction ____ clean lips ____ lateralization ____ midline-side ____ side; midline-side ____ side-side	____ anticipatory open mouth ____ jaw gradation ____ anterior bite ____ lateral bite ____ reduced strength of jaw closure ____ jaw thrust ____ tonic bite reflex ____ clenching ____ bruxism ____ anterior munching ____ straight munching ____ diagonal chew ____ rotary chew ____ bite/grind	____ delayed trigger pharyngeal swallow ____ absent trigger pharyngeal swallow ____ swallows per bolus ____ wet vocal quality before swallow ____ wet vocal quality after the swallow ____ cough before swallow ____ cough during swallow ____ cough after swallow
	Comments:			

Form 3–3. The Neonatal Oral-Motor Assessment Scale (NOMAS®)

Jaw		
Normal	**Disorganization**	**Dysfunctional**
____ consistent degree of jaw depression	____ inconsistent degree of jaw depression	____ extremely wide excursion that interrupts the intra-oral seal on the nipple
____ rhythmical excursions	____ arrhythmical jaw movements	____ minimal excursion; clenching
____ spontaneous jaw excursions occur upon tactile presentation of the nipple up to 30 minutes prior to a feed	____ difficulty initiating movements: ____ inability to latch on ____ small, tremor-like start-up ____ does not respond to initial cue of nipple until jiggled	____ asymmetry; lateral jaw deviation ____ absence of movement (% of time)
____ jaw movement occurs at the rate of approximately one per second (half the rate of NNS)	____ persistence of immature suck pattern beyond appropriate age	____ lack of rate change between NNS and NS (NNS = 2/sec; NS = 1/sec)
____ sufficient closure on the nipple during the expression phase to express fluid from the nipple	____ under 40 weeks PC (transitional suck)	

Tongue		
Normal	**Disorganization**	**Dysfunction**
____ cupped tongue configuration (tongue groove) maintained during sucking	____ excessive protrusion beyond labial border during extension phase of sucking without interrupting sucking rhythm	____ flaccid; flattened with absent tongue groove
____ extension-elevation-retraction movements occur in anterior-posterior direction	____ arrhythmical movements	____ retracted; humped and pulled back into oropharynx
____ rhythmical movements	____ unable to sustain suckle pattern for two minutes due to: ____ habituation ____ poor respiration ____ fatigue	____ asymmetry; lateral tongue deviation
____ movements occur at a the rate of one per second		____ excessive protrusion beyond labial border before/after nipple insertion with out/down movement
____ liquid is sucked efficiently into the oropharynx for swallow	____ incoordination of suck/swallow and respiration which result in nasal flaring, head turning, extraneous movements	____ absences of movement (% of time)

Form 3–4. Procedures for Conducting Pediatric Videofluoroscopic Swallow Study

Positioning: *Premature or small infants:* small Tumbleform™ seat with appropriate support for the trunk, neck, and head (45° angle).

Infants: medium or large Tumbleform™ seats, or MAMA™ (Multiple Application Multiple Articulation) seating systems.

Lead blankets should be used to shield the child below the waist.

Materials: Caregivers may be asked to provide any of the following that are regularly used at home. You should also have these on hand so you can try different utensils for therapeutic intervention.

1. A variety of nipples (preemie, regular, low flow, Haberman™)

2. A variety of cups, one possibly with a flow-guard lid

3. A variety of straws

4. Spoons of different sizes and bowl shapes (shallow vs. deep)

5. Syringe (Not ideal. Use cautiously.)

6. Pacifier

7. Liquid (glucose or formula, no breast milk)

8. Thickener

9. A sampling of the child's easiest/hardest foods across consistencies

10. Thick/thin pureed consistencies (pudding, applesauce)

11. Hard/soft solids (bread, vanilla wafer)

12. Liquid and paste barium

Presentations:

Infants

1. Liquid barium presented via syringe/spoon (2 ml).

2. Alternate NS (bottle) with NNS (pacifier).

Older Children

1. Begin with the easiest food mixed with barium and progress to the hardest.

2. Disguise barium in regular food.

3. If possible, test all food consistencies.

4. Try to make the examination as "normal" as possible:

   ❏ Fast-food packaging

   ❏ "You're trying my new recipe. Tell me how you like it."

Information Obtained

Oral Preparation/Oral Stage Bottle Feeding:

Normal

❏ immediate initiation to latch on

❏ immediate suck(le) onset

❏ nipple hold (posterior)

❏ tongue cupping around nipple

❏ strong lip/tongue seal

❏ stripping the nipple

❏ normal mandibular excursion

❏ rythmical sucking pattern

❏ burst is >30 seconds

❏ 1 or 2:1 suck/swallow ratio

Disordered

❏ decreased initiation to latch on

❏ suckle lag _____ (seconds)

❏ nipple hold (anterior)

❏ reduce tongue groove

❏ reduced lip/tongue seal

❏ difficulty stripping nipple, minimal fluid expression

❏ limited mandibular excursion

❏ arythmical or disorganized sucking pattern

❏ burst cycle is < 30 seconds _____

❏ > 2:1 suck/swallow ratio _____

Oral Preparation/Oral Stage: Spoon/Solid Feeding

Normal

❏ bolus formation

❏ bolus manipulation (lateral)

❏ bolus hold

❏ age-appropriate mastication

❏ normal lingual motility

❏ normal tongue tip elevation

❏ oral transit time < 1 second

❏ no residue

Disordered

❏ disorganized tongue movements resulting in reduced formation and manipulation

❏ reduced tongue motility

❏ reduced hold

❏ immature mastication pattern

❏ premature spillage into pharynx

❏ reduced control of a cohesive bolus

❏ reduced tongue tip elevation

❏ tongue thrusting pattern

❏ jaw thrusting

❏ piecemeal deglutition

❏ prolonged OTT _____(seconds)

❏ % residue _____ where _____

continued

Pharyngeal Stage

Normal

❑ triggering of pharyngeal swallow above vallecula (infants),

❑ triggering of pharyngeal swallow at anterior faucial arches (older children)

❑ velopharyngeal port closure

❑ adequate laryngeal elevation/closure

❑ adequate cricopharyngeal dilation

❑ adequate pharyngeal contraction

Disordered

❑ _____ (seconds) delay in triggering swallow response

❑ nasopharyngeal reflux

❑ reduced epiglottic inversion

❑ reduced laryngeal elevation/closure

❑ reduced cricopharyngeal dilation

❑ reduced pharyngeal contraction with residue

❑ _____% residue where _____

❑ _____% aspiration, when? (circle) before during after

❑ location of aspiration _____

❑ response to aspiration _____

Esophageal Phase

Normal

❑ normal esophageal transit

Abnormal

❑ reflux describe (where and how much) _____

❑ emesis

❑ stricture

❑ pain/agitation

❑ reduced peristalsis

❑ TEF

❑ obstruction

Recommendations

Diet

❑ NPO

❑ PO with enteral support

❑ PO feedings with special utensils

❑ Bolus size

❑ Control rate

❑ Control amount

❑ Solids

❏ Liquids

❏ Alternate liquids/ solids

❏ Liquid assist

❏ Nothing to eat/ drink within 2 hours of bedtime

Positioning

❏ Chin tuck

❏ Body position

❏ Turn head right/left

❏ Tilt head right/ left

❏ Provide support for jaw, lower lip, cheek

❏ Keep patient upright after meals

Strategies

❏ Altering the consistency, temperature, volume, and taste of food

❏ Changing feeding utensils/altering the nipple

❏ Multiple swallows

❏ Throat clearing

❏ Adaptive equipment

❏ Encourage AP movement of bolus

❏ Encourage lip closure

❏ Encourage chewing

❏ Check pocketing left/right

❏ Provide perioral nonnutritive

❏ intraoral stimulation before feeding

❏ Give frequent breaks during feeding

❏ Present food to right/left side of mouth

❏ No straws

❏ Provide distraction-free environment

❏ Terminate feedings

❏ Exhibits clinical signs of aspiration

❏ Deflate trach cuff during PO intake

❏ Suction before/after meals

❏ Check food in right/left cheek after meal

❏ Patient requires 1:1 supervision

Referrals

❏ Otolaryngology

❏ Gastroenterology

❏ Neurology

❏ Prosthodontics

❏ Dentistry

❏ Cardiology

❏ Other: _____

SECTION

THERAPY FOR FEEDING AND SWALLOWING PROBLEMS

● ●

This section outlines current treatment strategies for infants and children with dysphagia. Each section is divided into four sections: WHO? WHAT? WHY? and HOW? The WHO? section gives examples of feeding/swallowing disorders that would likely warrant the interventions described. Remember that these categories should not be considered as exclusive. Certainly, there are infants/children who present with unique feeding/swallowing problems not presented that may profit from these interventions.

TREATMENT STRATEGIES

In general, therapy can be divided into two groups: (a) compensatory strategies, which help to ensure successful feeding in the presence of the underlying disorder and (b) facilitative strategies, which promote and/or develop normal feeding skills.

Compensatory Strategies

- Establishing Optimal Infant State/Feeding Readiness
- Organizing the Infant for Oral Feeding/Altering the Environment
- Establishing Optimum Position
- Altering the Consistency, Temperature, Volume, and Taste of Food
- Changing Feeding Utensils

Facilitative Strategies

- Establishing a Nonnutritive Suck
- External Pacing/Establishing Internal Rhythm
- Oral Stimulation Program
- Reducing Oral Aversions
- Developing Chewing Skills
- Intervention for Behavioral Feeding Disorders
- Oral-Motor Therapy

The primary goals of dysphagia therapy are to promote adequate nutrition/hydration and develop age-appropriate feeding skills. No one way will work with every infant. Therapy must be customized to meet the individual needs of each child and consider the whole child within the context of her or his environment rather than focused exclusively on successful swallowing of food. Ultimately, the goal of therapy is to educate, train, and work collaboratively with the individual(s) who are primarily responsible for the development of the child within her or his family system. Table 4–1 summarizes common feeding problems, therapy suggestions, and goals.

TABLE 4–1. Typical Feeding/Swallowing Problems, Therapy Suggestions, and Treatment Goals

Problem	Therapy Suggestions	Rationale/Goals
Reduced extraction of liquid from the nipple, weak suck(le)	• Change nipples. • Establish and strengthen NNS. • Provide external jaw/cheek support. • Lingual stroking • Negative pressure	To increase liquid extraction from the nipple
Suck(le) lag	• Establish optimal infant state. • Establish NNS. • Organize the infant for oral feeding. • Provide lip and jaw support.	To increase initiation of nutritive suck(l)ing when nipple is presented
Disorganized suck(l)ing	• External pacing • Alter the nipple: slow the flow rate. • Establish an NNS. • Organize the infant for oral feedings.	To establish sustained, rhythmical nutritive suck(l)ing

Problem	Therapy Suggestions	Rationale/Goals
Anterior loss of food from mouth	• Jaw tapping • External lip/jaw support	To increase muscle tone and external support and facilitate retention of food within the oral cavity
Jaw thrusting	• Change feeding positions. Try head slightly reclined. • Provide jaw support. • Provide sensory stimulation. • Have the child practice holding objects between teeth.	To reduce jaw thrusting during feeding to improve oral preparation of food
Jaw retraction	• Provide jaw support as you manually pull jaw forward. • Change feeding position. Try head/trunk slightly inclined (forward).	To facilitate jaw extension during feeding to improve oral preparation of food
Jaw clenching	• Apply firm pressure to face and cheeks. • Hold mandible with palm of hand and provide external support. • Change feeding position. Try head/trunk slightly inclined (forward).	To facilitate graded jaw movements for food acceptance
Tonic bite reflex	• Apply firm pressure to face, cheeks, and gums. • Sensory stimulation to cheeks, lips, and chin. • Release the bite, apply bilateral pressure to the temporomandibular joint (TMJ). • Alter utensils (avoid utensils that can shatter or break). Try a flat bowled spoon (maroon spoon).	To reduce and manage the occurrence of the tonic bite reflex during feeding
Jaw instability	• Provide jaw support. • Provide sensory stimulation (cheek tapping). • Have the child practice holding objects between the teeth. • Alter feeding position (inclined, reclined, or upright) to determine which position optimizes jaw stability.	To facilitate graded jaw movements for food acceptance
Lip retraction	• Facial molding • Tap cheeks starting at the nose and moving to the upper lip. • Alter feeding position. Try head slightly flexed with loose chin-down position.	To promote lip closure during feeding

continued

TABLE 4–1. *(continued)*

Problem	Therapy Suggestions	Rationale/Goals
Reduced upper lip movement	• Begin at the middle of the upper lip and firmly stroke (3–5 times) to the corner of the mouth. Repeat on other side. • Same as above but tap • Alter the utensils. Try a straw. • Avoid scraping food from the spoon with child's upper teeth. Encourage lip closure around the spoon.	To faciliate upper lip movement for feeding
Low cheek tone	• Rhythmic tapping on the cheeks and TMJ • Facial molding • Cheek support • Alter utensils: Try a straw.	To increase muscle tone of cheeks and decrease loss of food in lateral sulci
Tongue bunching	• Alter feeding position: Try chin-down position. • Tap on dorsum of tongue and under base of chin. • Establish an NNS before feeding.	To flatten tongue blade in preparation for food manipulation
Tongue retraction	• Alter feeding position. Try head slightly flexed with loose chin-down position. • Establish NNS before feeding. • Rhythmic tapping under base of chin • Firm stroking of tongue starting at center and moving laterally in quick rhythmic stokes • Alter feeding utensil: Try a longer nipple.	To extend tongue anteriorly in preparation for food manipulation
Tongue protrusion/thrusting	• Change feeding positions. Try head slightly reclined. • Firm, downward pressure on center of tongue • Tongue tapping • Facial molding • Cheek support	
Reduced tongue movements (lingual hypotonia, reduced oral sensitivity, increased oral transit time and oral residue)	• Tongue stroking/tapping • Cheek support • Oral stimulation program • Pacing	To increase tongue motility and facilitate bolus formation, manipulation, and improve oral transit of food

Problem	Therapy Suggestions	Rationale/Goals
Nasopharyngeal reflux	<ul><li>Alter feeding position. Try head slightly flexed.</li><li>Alter the nipple: Reduce the flow rate.</li><li>Alter the consistencies of food: Try thicker liquids and foods.</li><li>Pacing</li></ul>	To reduce the occurrence of nasopharyngeal reflux
Delay in triggering the swallowing response	<ul><li>Thermal stimulation</li><li>Alter the nipple: Reduce the flow rate.*</li><li>Altering the consistency, temperature, volume, and taste of food*</li></ul>	To reduce aspiration risk by increasing the timing of the swallowing response
Aspiration during the swallow	<ul><li>Alter feeding position. Try head slightly flexed with loose chin-down position.*</li><li>Alter the utensil: Try an angle-neck bottle.*</li><li>Alter food consistency: Try thicker liquids/foods.*</li></ul>	To reduce the risk of aspiration during oral feedings
Aspiration after the swallow	<ul><li>Pacing. Allow for dry swallows to clear possible pharyngeal residue.*</li><li>Alternate food consistencies.*</li></ul>	To reduce the risk of aspiration after the swallow

*These therapeutic interventions should be tried during the VFSS to verify their effectiveness in reducing aspiration risk. You should never proceed with oral feeding if you suspect aspiration. A VFSS should be used to determine the safety of swallowing with the precautions.

Establishing Optimal Infant State/Feeding Readiness

WHO? Premature infants, older children with feeding disorders who are easily distracted or not responsive to feeding, infants/children who are disorganized, and infants/children with a weak suck.

WHAT? Apply alerting or calming techniques one at a time with the purpose of bringing the infant into an organized calm state. The principle behind the alerting techniques is to be arrythmical and to heighten the infant's state of attention. Use calming techniques to help organize and focus the infant before feeding.

WHY? To establish optimal state in which the infant is most alert and/or receptive to feedings (see Tables 1–5 and 1–6 on pp. 9 and 10, respectively). Infants and children must show responsiveness and signs of "readiness" before oral feeding can be established.

HOW? From Klein & Delaney, 1994; Wolf & Glass, 1992.

Calming Cues	Alerting Cues
Swaddle the infant to provide a firm and deep pressure and stability	Provide light touch/tickles to soles of the feet and palms
	Change the diaper before feeding
For older children use a calm, rhythmical rocking motion. For premature children, avoid extraneous movements.	Use a cold cloth (if medically tolerated)
Provide deep pressure to arms, legs, and trunk	Provide arrhythmical movement, gentle tapping, alter directions
	Gently rock the infant side to side
Provide quiet and unchanging environment	Allow a changing visual environment
Dim lights, neutral color	Bright lights, bright colors or contrast of color and shape, moving objects
Use either no noise or try white noise, quiet 4 × 4 beat music, repetitive noise	Allow for arrhythmical or unexpected noises or exciting music
Talk quietly to the infant in a monotone voice or do not talk at all	Talk in fluctuating pitch and loudness
Be predictable	Be unpredictable
Use bland-tasting food, smooth textures, neutral smells	Use bold-tasting foods (spicy, tart) with more texture, strong smells

Organizing Infant for Oral Feeding/Altering the Environment

WHO?	Infants who have a disorganized sucking pattern, premature infants, infants with state-related feeding disorders.
WHAT?	Getting infants organized so they are ready for oral feeding.
WHY?	To prepare the infant for feeding, prolong feeding endurance, and reduce the risk of aspiration.
HOW?	See below.

1. Feed the infant in a calm and quiet place. Eliminate all noises except for those that may have a calming effect on the infant.

2. Establish an external rhythm such as classical four-quarter time music, metronome, or other items that have quiet, repetitive sounds.

3. Dim the lighting.

4. Reduce the number of or eliminate visual objects and individuals located in the infant's field of vision.

5. Swaddle the infant in a blanket, providing gentle pressure.

6. Rock the older infant slowly before presenting the bottle.

7. Present the infant opportunities to suck on fingers and thumbs before the bottle is presented.

8. With a finger or pacifier, establish a paced NNS before presenting the infant with the bottle.

9. Avoid distracting movements by the feeder. Try not to stimulate the infant by giving chin support or touching the face unless necessary.

10. Feed the infant in a side-lying position. Some infants who do not tolerate handling are able to eat more safely with less physical exertion when laying on their side during feedings.

11. Change the feeding position. If the infant is supported well, a face-to-face hold will help the feeder monitor the infant's response. If the infant is disorganized, a cradle hold will provide more support and organization.

12. Watch closely for signs of emerging stress during and after feeding. Signs of stress during nipple feeding are presented below with the possible cause and solution (adapted from Shaker, 1998, and Wolf & Glass, 1992).

Signs of Stress	Possible Cause	Possible Solution
A subtle color change occurs over the course of the feeding.	Progressive oxygen desaturation caused by feeding the infant too fast.	Impose periodic breaks during the feeding.

Signs of Stress	Possible Cause	Possible Solution
A sudden change in color occurs during the feeding.	The infant may be "breath holding" during the feeding in response to a fast flow rate nipple.	Use a slow flow rate nipple.
A previously calm infant becomes fussy during feeding.	Fussiness is one of the first signs that an infant is losing control and becoming disorganized. The infant may be exhibiting difficulty completely protecting his or her airway (microaspirating).	Stop the oral feeding and reestablish the infant state.
The infant gets drowsy or falls asleep toward the beginning or middle of the feeding.	The infant may be exhibiting respiratory fatigue, general fatigue, and/or inadequate oxygenation. Sleeping may be the infant's way of "shutting down."	Stop the feeding. Allow the infant to rest then restart the feeding using pacing and frequent breaks.
The infant shows signs of respiratory distress: tachypnea, nasal flaring, chin up with neck extended position (chin tugging), shallow "catch up breaths" between suckle bursts, and high-pitched crowing sounds.	The infant is becoming disorganized and is having trouble protecting the airway. Chin tugging is one way to open the pharyngeal airway. The high-pitched sounds reflect incoordination of vocal fold opening/closing with respiration.	Stop the feeding. Allow the infant to rest then restart the feeding using pacing and frequent breaks.
The infant shows swallowing stress signals such as excessive drooling, gulping, multiple swallows, coughing, or choking.	Drooling may be caused by loss of control of the bolus. Gulping occurs when the infant uses a prolonged sucking pattern without adequate "catch up" breaths. Gulping and multiple swallows can also be signs that the infant is trying to feed too vigorously. Coughing or choking may indicate that liquids have entered the airway.	Drooling can be managed by allowing fewer sucks with pacing. Slowing the flow rate can help reduce gulping, multiple swallows, and coughing. Before restarting the feeding, allow the infant to self-regulate. If the infant does not regain color and respiratory status following a coughing episode, then intervention may be necessary.

Establishing a Nonnutritive Suck

WHO? Premature infants, infants who are disorganized, and tube-fed infants beginning an oral stimulation program.

WHAT? Nonnutritive sucking on a pacifier, finger, and/or thumb.

WHY? Nonnutritive sucking is a prerequisite to nutritive sucking; this will help establish a strong nutritive suck, making oral feeding possible. Nonnutritive sucking also improves weight gain in premature infants.

HOW? See below.

❖ Place a gloved finger or a pacifier in the infant's mouth.

❖ Press firmly 4–6 times (1–2 times per second) on the middle of the tongue.

❖ Pause to see if the infant continues unassisted sucking.

❖ Repeat as tolerated.

External Pacing/Establishing Internal Rhythm

WHO?   Infants who have poor suck-swallow-breathe coordination, children who have been documented to take multiple swallows per food presentation, and infants/children with poor feeding endurance.

WHAT?   For infants, the feeder establishes the safest number of suck-swallow-breathe sequences before expected fatigue and stops the feeding to allow the infant to rest. For older children, increase the time between food presentations to allow for subsequent dry swallows and pharyngeal clearance.

WHY?   This allows infants with poor suck-swallow-breathe coordination additional time breathing and decreases the risk of oxygen desaturation because of fatigue. Also, children requiring multiple swallows need additional time in order to reduce the risk of aspiration. This allows the feeder to manipulate the time between food presentations. Pacing can increase the child's success and interest in feeding.

HOW?   From Shaker, 1998.

❖ **If the Presentation Is Via a Bottle**

1. Present the bottle and let infant begin feeding.

2. Allow the infant to bottle feed for the prescribed amount of time (measured in seconds or number of suck-swallow-breathe cycles as indicated on the VFSS). Infants under 35 weeks typically display an immature suckling pattern (3–5 sucks per swallow).

3. After the prescribed time or numbers of sucks, tip the bottle down. If you need to break the infant's suction by pulling the bottle out of the infant's mouth, leave the nipple in contact with the infant's lips so the infant is cued that the feeding will continue.

4. Allow the infant to return to his or her baseline breathing.

5. Present the bottle again.

6. Repeat steps 1–5.

❖ **If the Presentation Is Via a Spoon**

1. Present the food to the child.

2. Allow the time to pass or the number of swallows to occur that was documented via the VFSS that was needed to adequately clear the bolus from the oral/pharyngeal cavities.

3. Present the food again.

Establishing Optimum Position

WHO?	All infants/children with feeding/swallowing issues should be fed in an optimal position. Changing the feeding position can greatly improve feeding/swallowing in infants with excessive jaw movement, a weak suck, and/or muscle tone issues.
WHAT?	Altering the positioning and posture of the infant or child to reduce the risk of aspiration and facilitate successful feeding.
WHY?	The position of the infant/child affects the stages of swallowing in addition to airway protection and respiration. Proper positioning is required to establish stability and mobility of the lips, cheek, jaw, and tongue. For example, if an infant's head is back, he or she will have less control of the oral structures because of decreased stability. The airway is more open, increasing the risk of aspiration. Older children whose muscle tone is hypertonic, hypotonic, or fluctuating often demonstrate poor trunk support with hyperextension of the neck, adduction of the scapula, and shoulder elevation (Morris, 1999a). These, in turn, affect head and neck control necessary for successful feeding.
HOW?	Compiled from Alexander, 1987; Schuberth, 1994.

❖ **Infants** (See Figure 4–1)

1. Head should be forward.

2. Neck elongation with the neck in a loose chin tuck position.

3. Infant's shoulders should be symmetrical and slightly depressed.

4. Hands should be drawn to midline.

5. Hips and knees should be flexed.

6. If needed, loosen the diaper to facilitate belly breathing.

7. Use a side-lying position for infants who do not tolerate being handled.

8. If the infant is well supported, use a face-to-face hold so that you can monitor the infant's response to feeding.

9. If the infant is disorganized, use a cradle hold to provide more support and organization.

❖ **Infants With Low Tone**

1. Keep the infant as upright as possible (45° angle). This will help the muscles to work harder and decrease the backflow of liquid into the ear canal (eustachian tube).

2. Rest only the head on your arm.

❖ **Infants With High Tone**

1. Slightly more neck flexion with chin tucked down.

2. Shoulders should be in a neutral position.

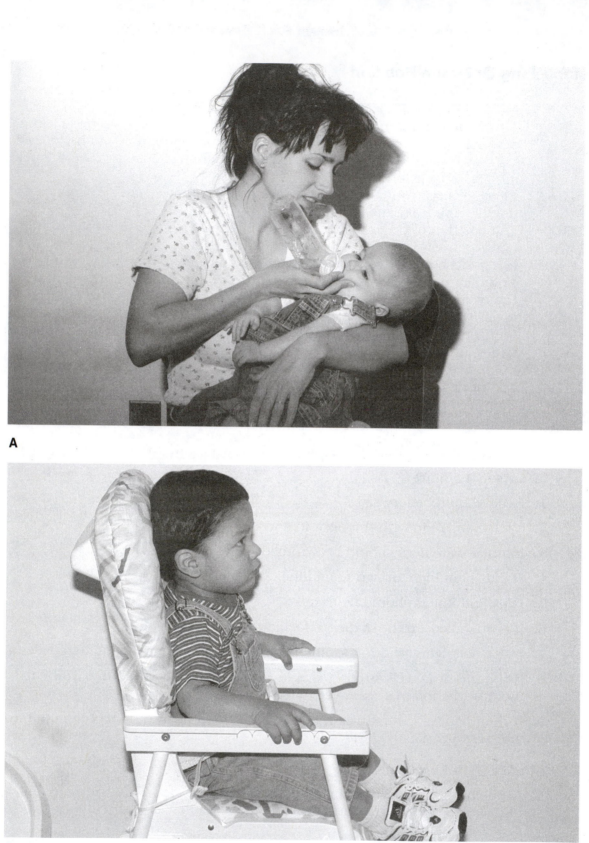

A

B

Figure 4–1. Examples of correct feeding positions for infants and children. **A.** Infant's shoulders symmetrical and slightly depressed, head forward, a loose chin tuck position, hands drawn to midline and hip and knees in flexion. **B.** child's head, neck, and spine are aligned over pelvis, and shoulders are back with proper hip flexion.

❖ Infants With GERD

1. Place the child at a 30° angle, prone upright position. Do this by elevating the head of the bed; do not use a car seat. This helps keep food away from the LES.

2. Keep the child quiet and in an upright, prone position for 30 minutes (or longer) after eating to allow for gastric emptying.

❖ Children With Poor Head and Trunk Control and Associated Problems
(e.g., jaw thrusting, retraction, instability or clenching, lip retraction, and tongue retraction)

1. Neck elongation with neck in a loose chin tuck position.

2. Trunk support through an adaptive seating system. Arms should be free to move.

3. Erect spine over stabilized pelvis.

4. Knees, feet, and pelvis are at 90° flexion.

5. Spine is perpendicular to the bottom of the seat.

❖ Children With Poor Head Control and Tongue Thrusting

1. A slightly reclined position may benefit the infant. (*Warning*: This makes the bolus harder to control in the oral cavity.)

2. Use towels or blankets to support the back in this reclined position.

Oral Stimulation Program

WHO?   Children who are NPO.

WHAT?   Stimulating the face and oral cavity with different textures, touch pressures, and temperatures.

WHY?   Providing the infant with oral stimulation helps to develop and/or maintain normal feeding development. The child will decrease her or his oral aversive behaviors when oral feeding is introduced.

HOW?   From Arvedson & Brodsky, 1993; Klein & Delaney, 1994; Wolf & Glass, 1992. See Figure 4–2.

❖ Provide the infant/child with opportunities to orally explore a variety of toys.

❖ Encourage the infant to suck on fingers and/or a pacifier during tube feedings.

❖ Rub the child's face with various textures (soft/smooth–stiff/rough).

❖ Use a finger to apply firm pressure to the gums, tongue, and teeth (if applicable). Start at midline and work your way back. Repeat 3–4 times.

❖ Provide the infant/child opportunities for NNS. In doing this you provide an infant opportunities to suck on an object (finger or pacifier).

❖ Provide the infant with a toothette, small NUK® toothbrush, or gloved finger dipped in water, formula, or breast milk. Apply pressure downward, and then apply a finger stroke. Repeat if the infant tolerates this and has a positive response.

❖ Modifying oral motor tone with sensorimotor techniques. For children with high muscle tone, use a soft cloth to apply deep, firm, rhythmic pressure around the mouth. Hold the child's cheek between your index and middle finger and shake the cheeks on both sides. This improves facial elongation. For children with low muscle tone, use light, rhythmic tapping and vibration to the cheeks. For either case, diagonal shaking of the tongue is reported to improve graded tongue movements and elongation. Firm, rhythmic tapping to the dorsum of the tongue reportedly improves tongue cupping (Alexander, Arvedson, Dorsey, & Pinder 1999).

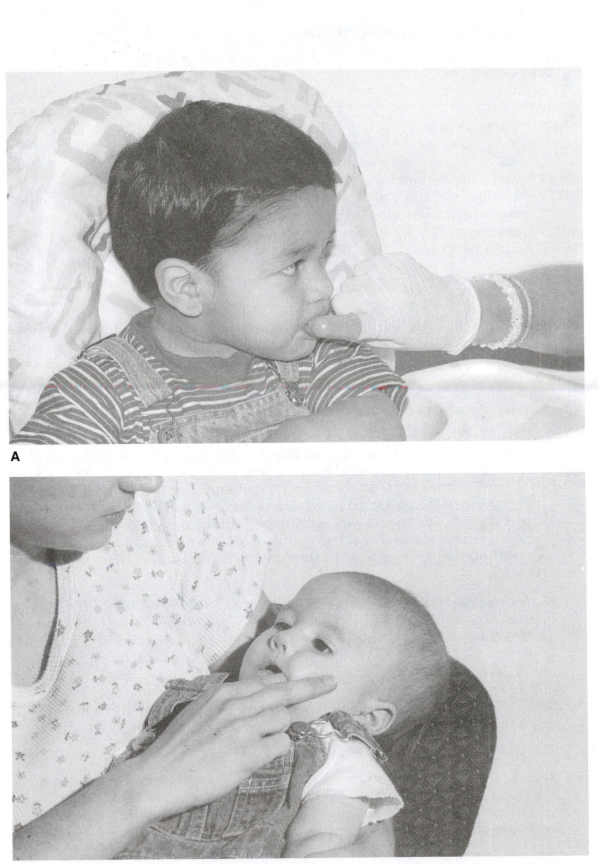

Figure 4–2. Examples of oral stimulation therapy techniques. **A.** Increasing sensitivity of lips using an Infadent®. **B.** Modifying oral motor tone. Here the mother is holding the child's cheek between the index and middle finger and shaking the cheeks on both sides to improve facial elongation.

Reducing Oral Aversions

WHO?	Infants/children with oral hypersensitivity (OFF, NOFTT), infants/children who have been previously tube fed, infants/children with a hyperactive gag, and premature infants.
WHAT?	Reducing oral aversions for feeding.
WHY?	To decrease the infant/child's oral sensitivity, increase tolerance of touch, establish positive oral experiences, and establish trust that is necessary for mealtime success.
HOW?	From Alexander et al., 1999; Morris, 1999b; Schuberth, 1994.

Starting points for children will vary. Some will not allow you near the facial area and others will have trouble tolerating external stimuli inside the oral cavity. If the infant/child has high muscle tone, carry out these techniques with deep firm pressure. If an infant has low muscle tone proceed with gentle tapping.

❖ **Starting Point Outside the Oral Cavity**

1. Begin by giving firm, deep pressure or patting to the part of the infant's body that is least sensitive. You may have to start with the hands and move up to the arms and shoulders before you can touch the face. Establish positive nonfeeding sensory experiences with the child. Therapeutic touch (pediatric massage) can be focused on the whole body, not just the mouth. This is especially important for the child who has had negative oral experiences. Follow the child's lead regarding what "feels good" and what does not. In this way, you establish a trust with the child.

2. Work your way gradually toward the face, continuing with the deep, firm pressure or patting that is rhythmic and predicatable. This will increase the child's tolerance to being touched.

3. When touch to the face is tolerated, start from the farthest point such as the ears or forehead and work your way toward the lips.

4. If the child becomes tense and uncomfortable throughout this progression, stop and reestablish a comfort level.

❖ **Starting Point Within the Oral Cavity**

1. Apply firm pressure to the outer part of the upper gum. Begin at midline and stroke in an anterior-posterior direction. Allow the child's cues to determine the rate and range of the stroking. Next, move to the lower gum and hard palate.

2. Using your finger, a familiar toy, tongue blade, NUK®, or spoon, press firmly (for children with high muscle tone) or tap gently (for children with low muscle tone) from the tongue tip, working your way back slow-

ly to the center and front of the infant/child's tongue. Avoid eliciting a gag. (See Figure 4–3.)

3. If possible, allow the child to hold your hand with the stimulus (toothette, NUK® toothbrush, soft toy) or use his or her own finger with your help.

4. If the child does gag, remove the stimuli and close the child's mouth.

5. Using a stimulus other than your finger, move from the center of the tongue to the anterior and lateral teeth/gums.

6. Give frequent breaks, because intraoral stimulation increases saliva production and the child will need to swallow more often.

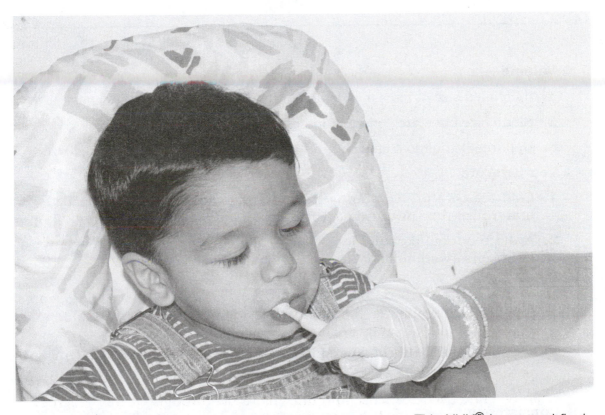

Figure 4–3. An example of one way to reduce oral aversions. This NUK® is pressed firmly (decrease tonicity) or tapped gently (increase tonicity) from the tongue tip, working back slowly to the center and front of the child's tongue.

Altering the Consistency, Temperature, Volume, and Taste of Food

WHO?   Infants/children who have a neurological impairment, infants with GERD, infants with a weak suck, infants/children transitioning from tube to oral feedings, and infants/children with sensory-based feeding problems.

WHAT?   Changing food presentation.

WHY?   If the child cannot cognitively participate in the feeding process, altering the presentation may compensate for the deficits and allow safe oral feeding. These techniques may help to decrease aspiration. For children transitioning to tube feedings, this helps to broaden the child's food repertoire and establish normal feeding development.

HOW?   See below.

❖ **Volume**

1. Increased size of bites may lead to a heightened sensory awareness.

2. Small size bites are generally indicated for oral stage deficiencies.

3. Document the most efficient and safe method during the VFSS.

❖ **Temperature**

1. Cold temperature can be used as alerting skills and provide a better oral transit time (Arvedson & Brodsky, 1993).

2. Avoid room temperature foods, especially liquids, as these provide the least sensory stimulation and may be more easily aspirated.

❖ **Taste**

1. Allow the child to taste strong flavors such as spicy, sour, or tangy.

2. Using a toothette, small NUK® toothbrush, gloved finger, and so forth, provide small tastes of different flavors (i.e., peppermint, salsa, lemon, salt, ketchup, pickle juice, barbeque sauce, hot sauces, cinnamon, nutmeg, etc.).

❖ **Consistency**

1. Make a list of the food types and consistencies that the child prefers. Work with the parents to determine what other foods within these categories can be introduced. For example, if the child has a preference for pureed consistencies limited to applesauce and creamed wheat cereal, work with the family or caregiver to determine what other foods within this category can be introduced next (e.g., pudding).

2. Expand foods within consistencies first and then begin to gradually increase or decrease the food texture to expand the food repertoire across categories. The following is a general description of various food consistencies.

- **Thin Liquids**

  Milk

  Water

  Carbonated water

- **Thickened Liquids**

  Applesauce in juice or milk

  Milkshakes

  Pudding in milk

  Yogurt in milk

  Juices with gelatin added

- **Strained/Pureed Foods**

  Solid, smooth foods that are pureed/blenderized

  Commercially available infant foods (avoid multiple consistencies)

- **Thickened Pureed Foods**

  Smooth but thick without lumps

  Gradually add crumbs from various crackers and cookies, bran flakes, wheat germ, and so forth

  Be aware of food allergies

  Add pureed fruit to juices

- **Lumpy Foods**

  Soft noodles, rice, canned pasta, mashed fruit (Stage 3 infant food)

- **Mashed Table Foods**
- **Chopped Solid Foods**

  Banana chunks, macaroni and cheese, chopped meatloaf

- **Whole Solids/Table Food**

Developing Chewing Skills

WHO? Infants/children who have neurological impairments, infants/children with GERD, infants/children transitioning from tube to oral feedings, infants/children with sensory-based feeding problems, and any infant who is having trouble moving from pureed to solid foods or refuses foods with texture (i.e., meats, vegetables, etc.).

WHAT? Assisting the child learning to masticate and manipulate new food textures without choking.

WHY? To expand the child's food repertoire and develop normal feeding skills.

HOW? From Klein & Delaney, 1994; Schuberth, 1994.

❖ Start by placing new soft solid textures (i.e., food strips of fruit, crackers, cereal) inside gauze that is tied tightly together with dental floss so you can pull it out if needed (sham bolus). Place food anteriorly on the tongue tip so the child can identify the food. Next, move the food laterally (on molars) to encorage tongue lateralization.

❖ Wrap chewy solid food strips (i.e., fruit snacks, meat, raw vegetables) inside gauze that is tied tightly together with dental floss. Place food laterally in mouth.

❖ Use external jaw support to assist with lip closure and graded jaw movements.

❖ Experiment with different food flavors (spicy, tart, sweet, sour) and temperatures (very cold to warm) to increase sensory input.

❖ Stroke up/down inside the cheek to promote chewing behaviors.

❖ Once the child is accepting and lateralizing food in gauze from midline of tongue to molars, introduce soft, soluble solids (i.e., crackers, cereal). Go slowly.

❖ Work on biting by placing cracker between lateral incisors and alternating sides. In addition to increasing biting stimulation, this may encourage the tongue to cross midline.

Changing Feeding Utensils

WHO?	Infants with oral stage problems caused by a variety of etiologies.
WHAT?	Altering the nipple in terms of size, shape, flaccidity, stiffness, and flow rates; try different feeding utensils.
WHY?	To establish optimal feeding success.
HOW?	From Arvedson & Brodsky, 1993; Klein & Delaney, 1994; Morris, 1997; Shaker, 1998; Tuchman & Walter, 1994.

1. **Nipples.** Table 4–2 describes some commercially available nipples and bottles.

   ❖ **Flow Rates**

   - The holes of a nipple should not be artificially enlarged. Nipples have 1 (slow flow) to 4 (fast flow) holes, are crosscut (fast rate), or single slot (variable flow).

   - Slower flow rates may be helpful for some infants with respiratory compromise, poor endurance, and weak suck. Single-hole nipples create a steady stream of liquid that may be easier to handle than bursts of liquid.

   - Faster flow rates may be helpful for some infants with intact pharyngeal swallow but early fatigue and some premature infants with higher suck-swallow-breathe ratios.

   - Dripless nipples (Haberman Feeder™) are ideal for infants who cannot hold small amounts of liquid in their mouth until they are ready to swallow. Instead of resting, they begin sucking again in response to the liquid, and this causes them to fatigue and become disorganized.

   - Preemie (red or blue) nipples tend to be crosscut with a faster flow rate. Preemie nipples were designed to deliver more liquid with less effort. However, the preterm infant's response to the faster flow is a faster respiratory rate. This can lead to fatigue and stress.

   ❖ **Stiffness**

   - The nipple should have enough stiffness to keep it inflated during sucking. If the nipple is too hard, the infant may tire easily. If the nipple is too soft, it may collapse during sucking and make the infant work even harder to draw fluid.

   - Children with hypotonic tongues may need a firmer nipple. Children with a weak suck or early fatigue may need a softer nipple.

   - Some nipples are designed with an antivacuum valve to prevent collapse during sucking.

TABLE 4–2. Commercially Available Nipples and Bottles

Product	Label or Manufacturer/ Distributor	Nipple/Bottle	Advantages	Limitations
Neonatal Nipple	Mead-Johnson Nutritionals Ross/Abbott Labs Wyeth	Smallest size Shortest shaft Single hole	Appropriate for very small preemies or infants with hyper-sensitive gag Temporary use prior to transitioning to longer nipple	Small shaft does not extend onto tongue to give sensory feedback Inappropriate for term adjusted-age infants
Premature Nipple	Mead-Johnson Nutritionals Ross/Abbott Labs Wyeth	Standard shaft Soft latex Single hole and/or cross-cut	Easy compressibility May help infant with low tone May be more sensitive to expression vs suction component of sucking	Rate of flow may be too rapid for infants with strong suck or high tone Nipple may collapse during sucking
Term Nipple	Several manufacturers and hospital suppliers	Standard shaft Single hole Latex or silicone	Size appropriate for most term adjusted-age infants Firmness provides sensory feedback to midline of tongue Easy commercial availability	
Cross-Cut Nipple	Johnson & Johnson Healthflow Newborn Mead-Johnson Cleft Palate Assembly Nipple Mead-Johnson Nutritionals Pigeon Bottle Nipple	Standard shaft[3] Long shaft[1,2,4] Latex[3] Soft latex[2,4] Silicone[1] Wide base[1]	Allows flow of thickened foods (1 tsp rice cereal to 1/2 oz fluid) No flow until baby sucks May assist infants with cleft palate[2,4]	Flow rate of thin liquids may be too rapid for some infants
Orthodontic or Nuk Nipples	Wyeth Mead-Johnson Nutritionals MAPA	Shaft angles toward posterior tongue and palate Single hole located at tip or top of nipple Wide base	Wide base may provide stability for infants with excessive jaw movement and inadequate jaw gradation Fast flow may assist term infants with low tone Inverting position of nipple may benefit some infants with cleft palate	Flow rate may be too rapid for infants with pharyngeal phase dysfunction or poor coordination Wide base may be too large for preemies Shape does not replicate breast nipple in mouth

Product	Label or Manufacturer/ Distributor	Nipple/Bottle	Advantages	Limitations
Playtex Natural Action Nipple	Playtex Products, Inc.	Small shaft Blunt nipple Wide base	Wide base provides deep pressure and sensory input to lips during sucking Nipple may extend and elongate like breast nipple	Latch-on and elongation of nipple are dependent upon a strong suck and central tongue grooving No evidence that air swallowing is reduced with bag insert Nipple and bottle work as system and are not interchangeable with other products
Grad-U-Feed Bottle	Mead-Johnson	Rigid 60 ml bottle with 1 ml gradations	Small bottle for infants requiring 2 oz or less than 2 oz of fluid	Bottle is too small for infants requiring more than 2 oz of fluid
Volu-Feed Bottle	Ross Labs		Volume consumed is easy to read Infant can maintain neutral or flexed head position	
Angled-Neck Bottles	Cherubs Comfortflow Corectro Corp. Degree Baby Products Johnson & Johnson (Healthflow) Natural Nurser	Shaped to angle fluid toward infant's mouth	Lessens tendency to tilt or hyperextend infant's neck as bottle is drained May reduce air swallowing Allows for neutral or flexed head position May reduce otitis media in some infants	Not critical for small infants who can use smaller bottles without excessive neck extension
Variable Flow Bottles/Nipples	Avent Bottle and Nipples/ Cannon Rubber, Ltd. Haberman Feeder/ Medula, Inc. Pigeon Bottle/ Pigeon Corp.	Horizontal slit rather than hole(s)[5,6] Flow rate limited by valve[6,7] Bottle compresses[7]	Horizontal slit allows for variable flow of fluid when manipulated by feeder[5,6] Nipple reservoir compresses[6]	Expensive Not available in retail stores; must be ordered from distributor Passive flow when overturned[5,7]
Compressible	Mead-Johnson Cleft Palate Nurser Pigeon Bottle/Pigeon Corp.	Soft, compressible	Enables flow when suck is ineffective (e.g., cleft palate)	Requires intact pharyngeal phase function Passive dripping from rim when bottle is compressed

[1]Johnson & Johnson Healthflow Newborn, [2]Mead-Johnson Cleft Palate Assembly Nipple, [3]Mead-Johnson Nutritionals, [4]Pigeon Bottle Nipple, [5]Avent Bottle & Nipples, [6]Haberman Feeder, [7]Pigeon Bottle.

Source: From Alper, B., & Manno, C. (1996). Dysphagia in infants and children with oral-motor deficits: Assessment and management. Seminars in Speech and Language, 17, 283–310. Reprinted with permission.

❖ Size

- The size should be appropriate for the size and shape of the child's mouth. If the nipple is too large or too long, it may cause gagging. If the nipple is too small, it may frustrate an older child.

- The "right size" nipple will allow the tongue to cup around it.

- Because preterm infants do not have fat pads, they may do better with a regular size nipple rather than a preemie nipple. The regular size nipple is larger and helps take up the room in their mouths, creating negative pressure for more efficient suckling.

❖ Shape

- The shapes of nipples vary greatly. Standard nipples are oblong and work well for children who can form a central groove.

- Flatter-shaped nipples are more breast-like.

- Nipples with a long, round cross section help to form a central groove.

- Long, thin nipples work well when the tongue is retracted by helping to bring the tongue forward.

- Wide nipples can be compressed to help with liquid extraction for children with cleft palate.

- Broad-based nipples can help create better negative pressure for sucking.

- Some nipples have a full or partial flap to cover a cleft palate (Brophy™ nipple).

2. Bottles

- ❖ Standard bottles hold 8 ounces (240 cc) of liquid. "Juice" bottles are smaller and hold 4 ounces (they also come with a crosscut nipple).

- ❖ The size and shape of the bottle should be easy for the infant and/or feeder to hold.

- ❖ Brightly colored bottles with designs provide visual stimulation.

- ❖ Angle neck bottles allow the infant to eat in a flexed or semiupright position. It is also good for the side-lying or prone positions.

- ❖ Soft bottles or bottles with collapsible plastic linings can be squeezed slightly to deliver liquid into the mouth.

- ❖ "Bubble-free" bottles have a vent at the bottom to allow air in.

- ❖ Haberman Feeder™/Mini Haberman Feeder™ are special bottle/nipple systems designed for children with craniofacial anomalies. The nipple is designed to accept 2 ounces of liquids and can be adjusted to three flow rates and a "no flow" rate. It allows for easy expression of liquid with minimal suction.

3. Cup

- ❖ Use a cup that can be tipped up to get liquid out but does not cause the child's head to tip backward (see Figure 4–4)

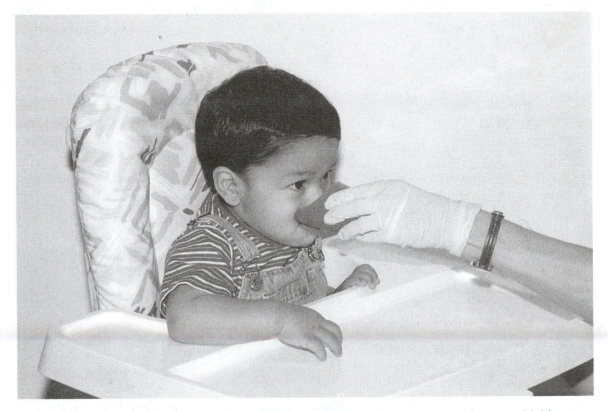

Figure 4–4. A flexible cut-out cup provides appropriate head positioning for cup drinking.

❖ Try using a sipper cup with a spout that supports adequate jaw and lip closure but does not cause the child to tip the head back to drink. Also, experiment with different types of spouted cups. Look for the one that provides the best control of the liquid flow relative to the child's ability to handle the volume of liquid presented.

❖ Only use cups that will not break, crack, or shatter if the child bites down on the edge.

❖ Ideally, the cup should be clear or opaque, allowing the feeder to observe the child's lips during drinking.

❖ Thick or rolled edges of a cup can provide extra stability for the child who needs to hold the edge of the cup with the teeth.

4. **Spoon**

❖ The bowl of the spoon should be relatively flat so that the child can remove food using the upper lip. Do not scrape food off the spoon with the child's upper teeth (see Figure 4–5). Also, the size of the spoon bowl should fit the child's mouth.

❖ The spoon should be hard enough so that it does not shatter or break, but pliable enough so that it will not damage teeth if the child bites down on it. Spoon bowls that are coated are also helpful for children who are hypersensitive to taste or temperature.

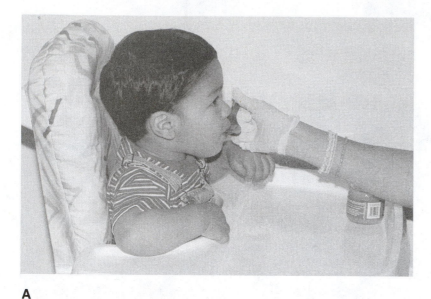

A

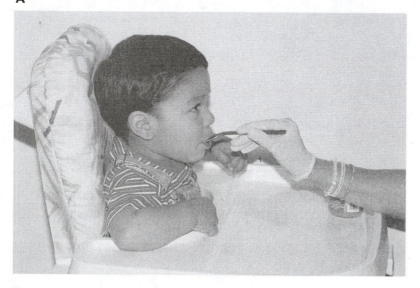

B

Figure 4–5. Examples of correct and incorrect spoon-feeding techniques. **A.** Side spoon feeding may help improve tongue lateralization. **B.** Correct spoon position for front feeding. Lips are closed around spoon, with slight neck flexion allowing for maximum lingual control of the bolus. **C.** Incorrect spoon position for front feeding. The child reacts by moving the chin upward thereby reducing lingual control.

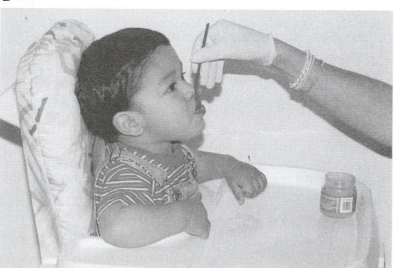

C

❖ When the child begins self-feeding, the spoon handle should be appropriate to the size of the child's hand (typically wide, thick, and short).

❖ The placement and pressure of the spoon in the child's mouth can also facilitate successful feeding.

Spoon Placement	Effect
Center of tongue with downward pressure.	Facilitates sucking movements and may help with posterior transit of the bolus.
Center of tongue with downward and inward pressure.	Encourages tongue movements up and down and reduces tongue thrusting.
Center of tongue, no pressure.	Promotes tongue movements forward and backward.
Alternating sides of tongue with light pressure.	Facilitates tongue lateralization and chewing.
Side of spoon presented to lips.	May help with tongue lateralization.

Intervention for Behavioral Feeding Disorders

WHO? Children who (a) are medically able to begin PO feedings and whose pharyngeal stage of swallowing is normal or children at low risk of aspiration and (b) demonstrate nonorganic failure to thrive (NOFTT) and (c) may present with an underlying oral motor disorder that makes them even more difficult to feed and/or (d) are fed orally but demonstrate oral aversive behaviors and a very limited food repertoire. Not all tube-fed children have difficulty transitioning to primary PO feeding, especially if they have received oral stimulation with nutritive stimulation. On the other hand, some children have extreme difficulty with this process and can be some of the most challenging therapy cases. Transitioning from tube to oral feedings, once medical clearance has been given, will most likely be a collaborative effort among the nutritionist, behavioral feeding specialist, and the speech-language pathologist or occupational therapist specializing in pediatric dysphagia.

WHY? To develop age-appropriate feeding skills and successful child/caregiver interaction. The oral stimulation program and reducing oral aversions, described previously, should be initiated before the child begins the transition to oral feedings in order to provide the child with positive sensory experiences involving the mouth area. Children who do not begin oral feedings before 12 months of age typically have a more difficult time developing normal feeding skills.

HOW? Adapted from Arvdeson, 1998; Babbitt, Hoch, & Coe, 1994; Morris, 1999a, 1999b; Palmer, 1993.

Treatment focuses on increasing appropriate feeding behaviors and decreasing inappropriate feeding behaviors. This focus will involve finding ways to motivate the child to demonstrate an already existing behavior more frequently (e.g., the child knows how to chew soft solids but is not motivated to do so) or teach the child feeding skills she or he does not already possess (e.g., the child has not been exposed to chewing soft solids before). The following is adapted from Babbitt et al. (1994).

Motivational Intervention

Increasing Desired Behavior

Find nonfood reinforcer (verbal praise, favorite toy, play, etc.). Whenever the child engages in the target feeding behavior (such as taking a bite), provide immediate positive reinforcement.

Decrease Undesired Behavior	Ignore inappropriate behaviors.
	Remove the reinforcer (i.e., in the case where feeding is usually terminated by the feeder if the child spits food, this reinforces the child to continue spitting. Instead, continue the feeding and re-offer the expelled food).
	Give positive reinforcement for other appropriate feeding behaviors.
Feeding Skill Acquisition	As you work to teach a child self-feeding skills, break the target behavior into small steps. Reinforce (shape) the desired behavior.

Arvedson (1998) presents "food rules" for caregivers that are basic to all young children (not infants) who are learning to increase their oral intake and/or are being introduced to new foods (adapted from Chatoor, Schaefer, Dickson, & Egan, 1984). These rules can be divided into three categories: scheduling rules, environment rules, and procedural rules. The following summarizes caregiver food rules:

- ❖ Maintain regular mealtimes; add planned snacks on a feeding schedule.
- ❖ Limit mealtimes to no more than 30 minutes.
- ❖ Do not allow the child to graze throughout the day. Only water should be presented between meals.
- ❖ Provide a neutral feeding atmosphere; do not force food or comment on the amount that was eaten.
- ❖ Protect the floor with a sheet and expect messes.
- ❖ No game playing. Never use food as a reward or present.
- ❖ Give small portions of solids first.
- ❖ Give liquids at the end of the meal.
- ❖ Encourage self-feeding (finger foods, utensil use).
- ❖ Remove the food after 10–15 minutes if the child is no longer eating or only playing with the food.
- ❖ Remove the food immediately if the child throws the food in anger.
- ❖ Reserve "clean up" for after the meal. Do not wipe the child's hands or mouth until the meal is finished.

Getting Started

1. Be sure the child is present at the table watching as other family members eat. This allows the child to experience the smells/sights of normal eating. Allow the child to smell, taste, and play with food. Make mealtime fun.

2. If the child is exclusively tube fed, get physician approval to begin bolus feedings (i.e., the child is fed via tube 3–5 times a day rather than continuously at night. This allows the child to experience hunger and normal stomach fullness). If possible, hold the infant in the same position during tube feedings as would occur if she or he were breast or bottle fed. Also allow the infant to nonnutritively suck during tube feedings to associate oral stimulation with the feeling of fullness.

3. Allow the child to mouth toys and utensils before presenting any food. See if the child will mouth foods that cannot be dissolved or swallowed for the tasting experience (i.e., beef jerky, hard licorice sticks) or mouthing toys that have been dipped in food for tasting (see Figure 4–6). The goal is to provide the child with positive oral experiences. Again, follow the child's cues and do not force the child to experience oral sensations.

4. If the child is also receiving oral motor therapy to improve feeding skills, this should be separate from mealtime.

❖ Introducing Food

1. Be sure that the child is hungry before beginning. Have the feeder (e.g., parent, caregiver) sit directly in front of the child and wait for him or her to show responsiveness.

2. Place small amounts of pureed foods on the child's lips. Use verbal cues like "Ready for a bite?" with the visual presentation of the spoon.

3. Reinforce successful feeding behaviors. If the child allows food to be placed in the oral cavity, give him or her positive reinforcement (verbal praise, access to a favorite toy).

4. Ignore inappropriate feeding behaviors.

5. Use a shallow-bowl spoon (see Figure 4–5B), and place pureed food consistencies in the center of the tongue to encourage anterior posterior movement. Thicker consistencies (e.g., ground) can be placed in the lateral sulci to encourage lateral tongue movement.

6. Go slowly. Allow the child to determine how fast or how much food to eat. However, be careful not to allow the child to feed too fast so that she or he is at risk for aspiration.

7. Mask new food tastes by mixing them wih preferred foods.

8. Gradually mix foods to alter textures, order of presentation, and portion size.

9. When beginning oral feedings, introduce different foods slowly to rule out allergic reactions.

10. Be patient. Allow 15–30 minutes for oral feedings, but do not make feeding punitive by keeping the child in the high chair for longer periods of time.

11. With the physician's/nutitionist's approval, use high-calorie food. Do not forget to include liquids. The child will never attain 100% oral feedings if she or he cannot maintain adequate oral hydration.

12. Chart oral intake for calories/amounts. Keep a food inventory. Treatment is likely to be successful if food preferences are used in conjunction with therapy.

13. For children who are transitioning from tube to oral feeding, note when the child is taking approximately half of her or his nutritional needs orally. Consider (with medical approval) a 60-hour wean. Here, tube feedings for caloric content are discontinued for 60 hours, and the child is fed orally exclusively. Use tube feedings only to maintain hydration.

14. The goal of all feeding therapy is a pleasurable experience associated with food. The first step is to determine if the problems are related to motivation or a skill deficit. The next steps are to increase appropriate feeding behaviors and decrease inappropriate behaviors.

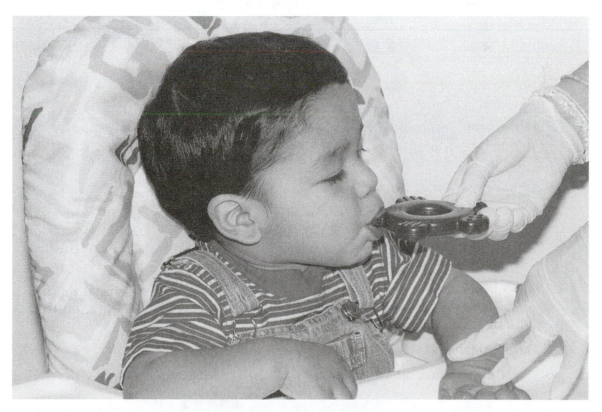

Figure 4–6. Presenting small tastes of food on a teether may help to facilitate the transition to spoon feeding by normalizing oral sensitivity.

Oral-Motor Therapy

WHO? Infants/children who show delays or deficits in feeding or nonfeeding oral movements.

WHAT? The establishment of oral movement patterns through sensory exploration, oral movement exercises to facilitate feeding skills, sound play, and speech development. This therapy focuses on increasing (or decreasing) oral tactile sensitivity, increasing (or decreasing) oral/facial tone, and stabilizing oral movements (i.e., jaw, tongue, lips).

WHY? Oral-motor therapy is designed to augment traditional articulation therapy by establishing "normal" oral movement patterns during feeding and nonfeeding activities that will, in turn, facilitate normal speech sound production. Although there continues to be controversy regarding the effectiveness of oral-motor therapy in the improvement of speech skills, the techniques employed to improve feeding skills have received less skepticism. Regardless of the lack of empirical support, clinicians working with children with feeding/swallowing issues appear to be willing to adopt new treatment approaches if they lead to faster functional outcomes. If, on the other hand, these approaches are not effective, then it is unethical to continue using these approaches (cf. Kamhi, 1999, for other factors that influence the selection of treatment options).

HOW? The focus of this section will be oral-motor therapy techniques (see Table 4–3) that may facilitate feeding skills.

TABLE 4–3. Oral-Motor Feeding/Swallowing Techniques

Technique	Rationale	Application
Chin and Lip Support	To improve jaw/lip stability	• Chin cupping: make a bowl shape with the entire hand and place it under the child's jaw with the thumb directly under the lower lip (see Figure 4–7). • Chin support with two fingers: place the index finger directly below the bottom lip and put the middle finger directly under the mandible. Place the thumb vertically along the side of the face. • Chin and lip support with three fingers: place thumb directly below the bottom lip, with middle and index fingers under the chin.
Jaw and Cheek Support	To improve jaw/cheek stability	• Place thumb under the chin with the index finger and middle finger on either side of the mouth (see Figure 4–8). • During bottle feeding, place middle finger and thumb on the infant's cheeks and apply firm support (see Figure 4–9).
Lingual Stroking	To increase tongue strength	• Place finger, spinning sucker toy, tongue blade, etc. on the midline of the tongue. • Stroke the tongue toward the front applying downward pressure. • Use quick, unpredictable movements • Tap to increase tone; use deep pressure to decrease tone.
Facial Molding	To relax the muscles of the cheek prior to feeding	• Use fingers or a warm, wet, or dry washcloth. • Begin at the periphery of the face (e.g., by the ears). • Work toward the chin and cheek, applying firm pressure toward the lip to obtain a closed mouth position. • Continue until you reach the mouth.
Cheek Tapping	To improve the infant/child tone	• Approximate the heels of your hand in a V position and cup the child's face. • Tap both sides of the child/infant's cheeks using firm but gentle pressure (if cheeks become red, adjust the pressure). • Do both cheeks simultaneously or alternately. • Do 10–20 times. • Use a NUK® toothbrush and roll it down the side of the cheek from the inside. • Utilize your index and middle finger.
Quick Stretch	To improve muscle tone	• Apply firm pressure with your fingers over the corner of child's lips and draw your fingers toward the child's cheeks. • Apply firm pressure to the masseter and buccinator muscles and draw your fingers toward the child's ears.

continued

TABLE 4-3. *(continued)*

Technique	Rationale	Application
Cheek/Lip Vibration	To improve tone	• Apply a commercially available vibrator to the child's cheek or lips. • Leave for 5–10 seconds. • Repeat.
Cheek Massage	To increase the tone of the cheeks	• Place your index finger inside the child/infant's mouth, middle finger across the cheek on the outside, then shake and vibrate the cheek gently (Figure 4–2). • Move the fingers toward the lips.

Increasing Tongue Mobility and Lip Closure	To establish labial and lingual movements necessary for diet advancement	• Before therapy, children need the following prerequisite skills:
		  1. Trunk control for sitting
		  2. The ability to hold the head up and turn it from side to side
		  3. The ability to close lips while food is in the mouth
		  4. The ability to move the tongue in and out
		  5. The ability to move the tongue up and down
		  6. The ability to keep the tongue inside the mouth while using it
		• *Tongue lateralization:*
		  1. Place small amounts of food between the cheeks and the tongue on lateral sides and have the child get it out.
		  2. Put a NUK® massage brush on the side of the tongue and roll it toward the cheek, which will stimulate the child's tongue to move in that direction.
		  3. Stroking the sides of the tongue may facilitate movement.
		• *Tongue tip elevation:*
		  1. Using a NUK® brush, Infa-dent®, or gloved finger, gently roll it into the child's mouth. Never push or force the mouth to open.
		  2. Press up and down on the dorsum of the tongue, maintaining tongue contact. Repeat for 10–30 seconds as tolerated. Increased times are associated with more saliva production that can pool in the mouth, providing the child with liquid to swallow.
		  3. Next, firmly press against the alveolar ridge, giving a tactile target for the tongue tip.
		• *Reducing tongue thrust:*
		  1. Place spoon with bolus on infant's tongue and press firmly down on tongue dorsum.

Technique	Rationale	Application
		• *Lip support/closure:*
		1. Start just above the upper lip. Gently press and follow the orbicularis oris muscle around the mouth.
		2. Next, use your fingers to manually close upper and lower lips or pull the cheeks forward.
Thermal Stimulation	Increase sensitivity	• *For older children:*
		1. Prior to feeding an infant, obtain a size OO laryngeal mirror or a small metal spoon.
		2. Chill the mirror/spoon in a cup of ice (use sterile ice chips if the infant is NPO/has an absent swallow).
		3. Stroke the soft palate and anterior faucial pillars. Go slowly to avoid eliciting the gag reflex. If possible, allow the child to place the spoon in his or her mouth.
		4. Do 10–15 times and instruct the child to swallow.
		• *For younger children:*
		1. Cold pacifier: drill a hole in the back side of the pacifier, fill with water, allow to freeze, and place pacifier in the baby's mouth. Remove the pacifier before the ice melts.
Negative Pressure	To promote a stronger lip/tongue seal for sucking	• Allow the baby to begin sucking on the bottle.
		• Gently begin to pull the bottle to the anterior part of the mouth while keeping the bottle in the infant's mouth.

Sources: From Arvedson & Brodsky, 1993; Alexander, 1987; Beecher, 1994; Klein & Delaney, 1994; Shaker, 1998; Tuchman & Walters,1994.

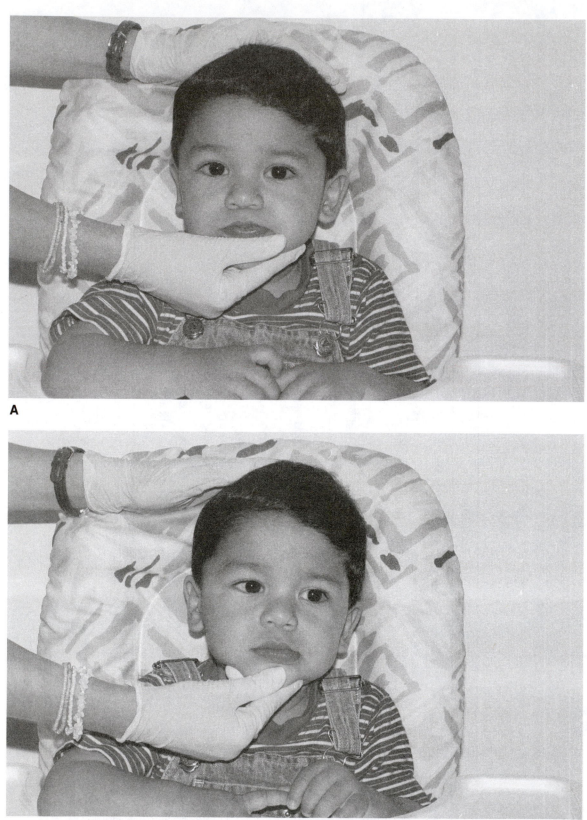

A

B

Figure 4–7. Examples of external chin and/or lip support. **A.** Chin cupping with lip support. **B.** Chin/lip support with three fingers.

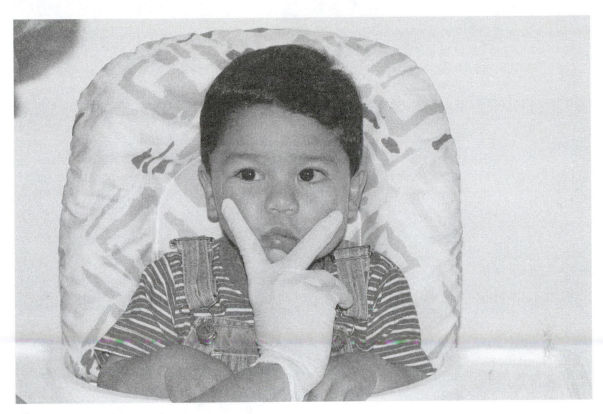

Figure 4–8. Jaw and cheek support.

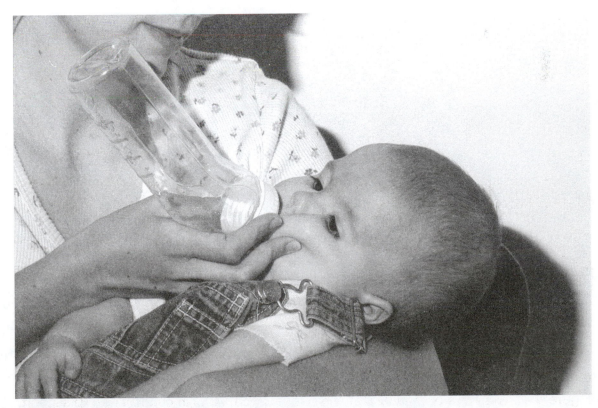

Figure 4–9. Cheek support during bottle feeding.

SECTION

CASE STUDIES

TOPIC I: GASTROESOPHGEAL REFLUX

Case 1

Child: Alex

Gestational Age: 35.5 weeks

History: Alex was born after an uncomplicated vaginal delivery. During feedings, Alex presented with episodes of apnea, oxygen desaturation, cyanosis, and frequent emesis. He demonstrated occasional stridor after feedings, followed by oxygen desaturation.

Results of Feeding/Swallowing Evaluation

Alex demonstrated good oral-motor control with mildly reduced coordination of the suck-swallow-breathe sequence. The suck-swallow-breathe ratio varied from 2:1 to 4:1 throughout the feeding. Episodes of gulp breathing and air swallowing were noted. When Alex was repositioned during feeding, he suffered apnea and subsequently became cyanotic with bradycardia. He was referred for further testing to rule out possible gastroesophageal reflux.

Results of Testing

Pneumogram: Mixed apnea and oxygen desaturation were found.

Technetium Scan: This procedure was completed to assess the presence of GERD. Results showed poor esophageal motility and pooling of liquid in the inlet of the stomach, followed by episodes of GE reflux, approximately half of which reached the oral cavity.

Treatment and Management

Alex was placed on an antireflux feeding plan that included upright positioning during feeding with thickened liquids. Antireflux medications were also prescribed.

Summary

Alex's symptoms, including apnea and the timing of the oxygen desaturation, were classic signs of GERD in premature infants. The presence of stridor associated with frequent emesis should also alert the clinician to a possible reflux disorder. This case illustrates how a clinical feeding evaluation can help in the early detection of GERD in premature infants, thereby reducing the risk of unnecessary medical testing.

Case 2

Child: Steve

Age: 18 months

History: Steve was delivered via cesarean section at 36 weeks. His mother described Steve as a "slow feeder." He was breast fed every 1½ hours and given a total of 8 oz of breast milk via bottle three times per day. During both breast and bottle feedings, Steve became agitated and would only take approximately 2 oz per feeding (or nurse for about 5 minutes at a time). His developmental feeding milestones were normal; however, his mother was concerned because Steve had a very limited diet, frequently refused to accept foods requiring mastication, and ate frequently but "never finished a meal."

Results of Feeding/Swallowing Evaluation

Steve presented with normal oral-motor and feeding skills. Because of his history of agitation during and after meals, snacking, and limited food repertoire, he was referred for further testing to rule out gastroesophageal reflux.

Results of Testing

Barium Swallow: Initially, a pH probe procedure was recommended to measure the occurrence of possible reflux over a 24-hour period. Steve's parents, however, were not receptive to the invasive nature of this diagnostic procedure and chose instead to try a barium swallow first. The barium swallow failed to show spontaneous reflux. However, when abdominal pressure was applied, reflux was noted to the level of the lower esophagus.

Treatment and Management

Steve was placed on an antireflux feeding plan that included small, frequent meals and upright position after feeding. Antireflux medications were also prescribed. He also participated in a feeding therapy program to reduce food aversions and expand his diet.

Summary

Given Steve's age, this conservative approach to GER management was tried first with the hope that over time the GER would resolve. Earlier identification of GER may have prevented his behavioral-based feeding problems. It was recommended that Steve be seen in 6 months for further GER testing.

TOPIC II: TRACHEOESOPHAGEAL FISTULA

Child: Hannah

Gestational Age: 1 day

History: Hannah was born full term after an uncomplicated pregnancy, labor, and delivery. Her vital signs and functioning were normal until 7 hours of life, when she was given her first bottle of glucose water. She started coughing, choking, gasping for air, and quickly became cyanotic. As a result, feeding was discontinued. Secondary attempts to feed were made at 11 hours of life. Oxygen therapy was utilized to lessen the degree of distress demonstrated on initial feeding; however, it was not effective. Coughing, choking, gasping for air, and cyanosis were again noted. Feeding was terminated and a standard upper-GI with videofluoroscopic swallow study was recommended to rule out aspiration.

Results of Testing

A type H tracheoesophageal fistula was discovered, causing consistent tracheal aspiration.

Treatment and Management

Surgery was required to close the fistula and divert the esophagus.

Summary

Esophageal stenosis may follow the surgical repair and cause continued dysphagia. Modifications to Hannah's diet and continued esophageal dilation may be necessary.

TOPIC III: PREMATURITY

Case 1

Child: Kari

Gestational Age: 34 weeks

History: Because of her mother's preclampsia, Kari was delivered via cesarean section at 26 weeks. At birth she weighed 1350 grams. She received positive pressure ventilation for the first 16 days, followed by supplemental oxygen therapy. At 30 weeks, nursing staff reported a possible seizure episode. She was referred for an MRI, which indicated an intraventricular bleed with significant pooling in the left lateral ventricle requiring a reservoir (needle aspiration). Her NG tube was replaced with a G-tube at 34 weeks. At this time, Kari was referred for a feeding evaluation to promote the development and maintenance of normal oral-motor feeding skills. She began an oral stimulation program to establish an NNS. Kari was discharged from the hospital at 38 weeks and was followed weekly through the oral-motor feeding clinic.

Results of Testing

Neurologic Examination: Mild-moderate right-sided muscle spasticity with oral-facial hypertonia were noted and presumed to be the result of the neurologic insult.

Summary of Feeding/Swallowing Evaluation: A clinical feeding evaluation revealed increased oral-facial tone resulting in abnormal movement of the jaw, tongue, and lips. A weak nonnutritive suckle was observed. NNS stimulation using firm, rhythmic pressure was provided before introduction of breast milk via bottle. Initial feeding was attempted using a Habermann feeder at a slow flow rate. Kari's suck-swallow-breathe coordination appeared adequate for the first 2 minutes with a 2:1 ratio. However, she fatigued quickly and pulled away from the nipple and coughed. A videofluoroscopic swallow study was conducted to rule out aspiration. Kari evidenced good coordination of suck-swallow-breathe during the first 2–3 minutes of feeding using the Haberman feeder at a slow flow rate. When she began to experience fatigue and stopped sucking, liquid collected in the vallecula and was eventually aspirated.

Treatment and Management

To compensate for her hypertonic posturing patterns that occurred during the feeding, Kari was repositioned to improve the alignment of the shoulders, neck, and head. This appeared to help reduce overall muscle tone. External jaw support during suckling, external rhythm, and pacing also increased the efficiency and duration of feedings. Firm pressure on the cheeks and around the mouth also promoted overall decreased tone. Facilitating a stronger suckling pattern required firm cheek and jaw support and a smaller bottle to allow the feeder to provide that support. Gently trying to pull the nipple out of Kari's mouth provided a slight traction on the nipple, which promoted stronger suckling. Increasing the bolus was effective in reducing the early fatigue, as Kari was able to coordinate swallowing and breathing with the larger size with less effort. Kari began to gain weight and grow at an appropriate rate for her condition.

Summary

Kari's feeding difficulties were a result of the neurologic insult incurred following an IVH. The neural damage caused a weak suckle and oral-facial hypertonia, which were managed through an oral motor program. Kari continues to grow and is now in the normal weight gain range for children her age. Although Kari has mild cerebral palsy, she continues to eat and develop without difficulties.

Case 2

Child: Haley

Age: 16 months

History: Haley and Kayla were monozygotic twins born prematurely at 23 5/7 and 24 1/7 weeks postconception age and weighed 950 grams (1 lb 5 oz) and 750 grams (1 lb 3 oz), respectively. Kayla survived only 11 days. Haley survived with aggressive treatment including high-frequency jet-ventilation and prolonged oxygen therapy. She subsequently developed bronchopulmonary dysplasia, retinopathy of prematurity, GERD, and grade 2 intraventricular hemorrhage. She received 12-hour continuous drip NG tube feedings and was placed prone in a sling to also help reduce episodes of reflux. She started an oral stimulation program at 32 weeks and began bottle feeding using a Haberman feeding system with a slow flow rate at 35 weeks. Her first feedings were successful; however, because of the energy she expended when feeding, the neonatologist suggested higher calorie formula feedings so that Haley could continue to gain weight. Haley continued to increase her oral intake and was discharged at 39 weeks. She received 4 ounces of formula four times a day and continuous drip NG tube feedings at night. At 3 months corrected age, her mother reported that Haley stopped oral feedings, became orally defensive, and stopped mouthing. A barium swallow study revealed GER, and Haley underwent a Nissen fundoplication with G-tube placement. She did not receive oral stimulation during this time and refused to nonnutritively suck. Because of Haley's distance from the medical center where she was born, she received outpatient feeding therapy twice per month. When she was referred to our facility, which was closer to her home, she was 12 months old, blind, orally defensive, and receiving 100% enteral nutrition. She did not mouth on toys or allow any sensory stimulation above the level of her shoulders.

Treatment and Management

Haley was seen at her home for weekly oral-motor feeding therapy. The therapist worked closely with a visual impairment specialist and the mother to determine what Haley's comfort zone for touch was and working up from that point to the face. Because of Haley's visual impairment, more verbal, auditory, and tactile cues were given so that she would feel control over what was happening to her. Her mother established a routine for Haley that included predictable mealtime experiences where Haley would sit in her high chair during family meals and play with food and utensils. Using an oral stimulation program, Haley slowly allowed firm touch to her cheeks and nonnutritive sucking on her thumb. She was encouraged to mouth toys and began a tasting program. Although she never accepted bottle feeding, Haley did accept small amounts of very thin cereal mixed with formula via spoon. Textures and amounts were gradually increased using behavior shaping and strong positive reinforcement. The biggest challenge was with cup drinking. Several different cups were tried but Haley had difficulty with lip closure around the cup or a spout. By 16 months she only accepted offered sips when a reward was offered (i.e., singing a favorite song after a sip, etc.).

Summary

Haley's case illustrates the importance of providing oral stimulation during the period when oral feeding is not possible. Haley did not receive oral stimulation therapy between 3 months to 12 months, a critical period for the acquisition of normal feeding skills. The result is a long-term behavioral feeding problem.

Case 3

Child: Connor

Gestational Age: 34 weeks

History: Connor was born premature at 29 weeks. He was on the ventilator for 4 days and received oxygen therapy for 1 week after that time (he was on a nasal cannula with a half liter of oxygen). Although there were respiratory concerns, Connor appeared neurologically stable. At 34 weeks oral feedings were begun. The nursing staff reported being uncomfortable feeding Connor because he desaturated and experienced bradycardia at least twice with each feeding. An oral-motor feeding evaluation was ordered to rule out aspiration and determine Connor's candidacy for continued oral feedings.

Summary of Feeding/Swallowing Evaluation

Connor demonstrated poor oral motor skills characterized by weak oral muscle tone and reduced tongue movements. His tongue was bunched and retracted. Inconsistent rooting behaviors were also observed. Connor became stressed before the assessment was complete. Saturation levels dropped to the low 90s when any stimulation was presented. Connor did not initiate a suck on a gloved finger, pacifier, or bottle. He presented with moderate baseline congestion that was heard clinically and through cervical auscultation. His nonnutritive suck was very disorganized, with short burst cycles of 1–4 and poor maintenance. Connor was presented with bottle feedings using a single hole nipple. His nutritive suck was very disorganized and lacked oral control. He immediately desaturated and was unable to sustain sucking. Because of his reduced endurance, therapeutic techniques could not be attempted. It was recommended that Connor receive primary enteral support with oral stimulation to facilitate a rhythmic NNS and increase feeding endurance. The neonatologist disagreed with the recommendations and ordered continued oral feedings. The nursing staff agreed to feed Connor by giving only one suck per swallow using a slow flow nipple, allow a rest break, and stop feedings after two desaturation episodes. The speech-language pathologist also provided oral-motor stimulation before feedings to help organize Connor. The parents were also trained, and all ideas/plans were posted bedside. Connor continued to stress during feedings, and the physician was again approached about the safety of continuing oral feedings. Although Connor was young, a videofluoroscopic swallow study was recommended to rule out aspiration. Once again the physician disagreed with the recommendations and ordered continued oral feedings. Connor received oral feedings for 2 days, after which time he went into respiratory distress and coded. Once medically stable, oral feedings were withheld and an oral stimulation program was implemented. Connor successfully began oral feedings at 36 weeks.

Summary

This case, unfortunately, illustrates how lack of communication among team members can lead to further medical problems. Because of the communication breakdown between the nursing staff, speech-language pathologist, and the neonatologist, Connor's transition to successful oral feedings was not only interrupted, but potentially life threatening.

TOPIC IV: CARDIAC DEFECTS

Case 1

Child: Matthew

Age: 3 months

History: Matthew was a full-term infant born to a healthy mother after a normal pregnancy, labor, and delivery. He was released from the hospital after 2 days. Breast feeding was progressing normally, and he was showing adequate weight gain at the time of dismissal. At the age of 3 months, Matthew began to feed poorly, often falling asleep before finishing the feeding. Matthew's father began feeding him breast milk with a Playtex® bottle/nipple system. His father was concerned that during bottle feeding Matthew was not breathing regularly and also commented that Matthew stopped breathing when he was crying. His pediatrician referred Matthew for a videofluoroscopic swallowing examination with follow-up esophagram because of his recent decline in weight gain.

Results of Testing

Videofluoroscopic Swallow Study: Matthew demonstrated a rhythmic and strong suckle that was efficiently coordinated with swallowing and breathing at the beginning of the feeding. His suck-swallow-breathe ratio was 1:1:1, and the suckling burst lasted approximately 45 seconds before he paused briefly to rest. As feeding progressed, however, coordination of suckling, swallowing, and breathing gradually worsened. In addition, sucking bursts were separated by increasingly longer respiratory pauses. Matthew eventually stopped feeding and fell asleep, most likely because of fatigue. He was referred for a cardiac evaluation.

Esophagram: An aortic vascular ring was found wrapped around the trachea. Increased activity and blood flow caused the tracheal restriction and subsequent reduced airflow during feedings.

Treatment and Management

Cardiac surgery was performed to correct the anomaly. Feeding improved slowly, returning to normal by 4 weeks after the surgery.

Summary

Sudden changes in feeding habits can indicate major medical problems in several body systems, including those that appear to have no relationship to feeding whatsoever. Matthew appeared to have normal feeding/swallowing skills. However, he experienced periods of apnea during feeding and crying (both of which are times of increased effort or activity), but not during sleep (a time of reduced activity). These symptoms suggest that something was occurring during feeding that was compromising Matthew's ability to breathe adequately while feeding. Because feeding and crying are the activities requiring a significant amount of energy expenditure that can tax the respiratory system, it is during these taxing times that the effects of tracheal compression were first noticed. As a result, Matthew rejected feeding in favor of breathing.

TOPIC V: NONORGANIC FAILURE TO THRIVE

Case 1

Child: Johnnie

Age: 6 months

History: At 3 months of age, Johnnie contracted a viral infection that resulted in a dramatic loss of appetite, emesis, and refusal to breast feed. His mother described his feeding during this time as "difficult." She switched to bottle feeding using a NUK® standard nipple and reported that although he resisted, she was able to "make him eat." During the time that Johnnie was ill, feeding was attempted every 1–2 hours. He cried during every meal, and his mother noted that feeding was a constant battle. In an attempt to continue providing nutrition for Johnnie, his parents reported they could successfully feed him with a bottle while he slept. After Johnnie recuperated from the viral infection, his aversion toward feedings became stronger. Feeding became such a struggle that his parents discontinued oral feedings during the day and would only feed him at night when he slept. Johnnie was 4 months of age and at the 15th percentile for weight when he was diagnosed as failure to thrive and referred by his pediatrician for a feeding and swallowing evaluation.

Treatment and Management

Intervention consisted of parent education and counseling, along with consultation with a nutritionist to increase Johnnie's caloric intake for wakeful feedings, as feedings during sleep were faded out. Johnnie's parents were instructed to create a calm and nonthreatening feeding environment for Johnnie and to discontinue feedings during sleep. An oral stimulation program was introduced, and Johnnie began nonnutritively sucking on a NUK® pacifier. He gradually began to accept a bottle, and his parents were educated regarding Johnnie's behavior cues to stop feeding. Two months postintervention, Johnnie's weight had increased to the 50th percentile. Bottle feeding was less difficult, and Johnnie had begun to accept cereal as well.

Summary

Johnnie demonstrated normal feeding development that was interrupted by an illness. Because he was force fed, Johnnie associated feeding with negative stimuli. Family counseling and education, as well as coordination with the nutritionist, were the keys to his continued feeding success.

Case 2

Child: Lauren

Age: 3 months

History: Lauren's weight at birth was 6 lbs 4 oz. At 4 weeks of age, her weight had dropped to 5 lbs. She was referred by her pediatrician to the oral-motor feeding clinic to determine the etiology of her suspected failure to thrive.

Results of Testing

Clinical Oral-Motor Feeding Evaluation: The mother reportedly breast fed Lauren regularly throughout the day. Lauren was the first child, and it was apparent during the interview that her mother had limited knowledge of "normal" weight gain and feeding patterns of infants. Lauren's mother reported that Lauren slept a lot during the day and through the night. She also commented that she felt uncomfortable waking Lauren to eat. Results of the clinical exam revealed normal oral-motor feeding skills; however, Lauren appeared to fatigue early during feeding.

Treatment and Management

Lauren's mother was counseled and educated regarding normal feeding schedules for infants, especially the importance of waking Lauren to maintain the feeding schedule. She was instructed to feed Lauren often during the day and to pace feedings so that Lauren would feed for about 5–10 minutes on one breast then rest for 5 minutes before feeding on the other breast. Lauren's mother was referred to the lactation specialist to address questions regarding breastfeeding techniques and lactose engineering. This involves pumping the lower calorie foremilk so that the infant nurses and receives the higher calorie hind milk. It was suggested that Lauren return to the feeding clinic every 2 weeks for a weight check. At 3 months of age, her weight had increased to the 50th percentile for her age.

Summary

Pacing feeding can be helpful for infants who have reduced endurance for a full feeding. Care must be taken not to overlook a possible medical condition causing the fatigue (such as cardiac problems).

TOPIC VI: MULTIPLE DISORDERS

Case 1

Child: Jamie

Gestational Age: 49 weeks

History: Jamie was born prematurely at 26 weeks gestation. He had a complicated medical history that included intrauterine drug exposure, Grade II IVH bilaterally (resolving), hydrocephalus with shunt placement, intensive antibiotic therapy for treatment of sepsis, NEC, and prolonged ventilation causing chronic lung disease. He was referred for a feeding evaluation at 35 weeks to assess the nature of his poor oral intake.

Results of Feeding/Swallowing Evaluation

A clinical feeding evaluation revealed reduced oral-motor skills. Oral movements were weak and slow but appeared adequate to support oral feedings. He demonstrated interest when presented with the bottle but evidenced difficulty coordinating the suck-swallow-breathe sequence (he was still on a nasal cannula) and fatigued quickly. He experienced inconsistent mild amounts of congestion but no coughing/choking, desats, or other signs of aspiration. After monitoring for a few weeks with no progress, a videofluoroscopic swallow study was suggested; however, the physician refused the study.

Treatment and Management

The speech-language pathologist continued to monitor oral feeding. Jamie made slow progress but was never able to take a full feeding orally. When the nurses would wean him from the nasal cannula, it was always put back on for feedings because of fatigue and effort needed. Because there was nothing else to offer, monitoring oral feedings was discontinued. New orders for a feeding evaluation were received approximately 4 weeks later. Jamie was still in the NICU because of decreased oral intake and refusal to eat. The nursing staff reported a possible sensory disorder because Jamie refused to eat after 15–30 cc. He enjoyed nonnutritive sucking and was noted to have a strong suck. Over the next week, his suck became weaker and he took 10–15 cc orally. A videofluoroscopic swallow study was recommended again at this time to rule out aspiration even though there were no obvious clinical signs. Again, the study was refused. Results of an MRI indicated a posterior fossa cyst. An ENT consult revealed tracheal malacia (trachea collapses during breathing). Because of protocol, all patients with a diagnosed malacia must have a videofluoroscopic swallow study because of risk of aspiration. The VFSS revealed poor expression of the liquid from the bottle and reduced control with vestibular penetration and aspiration (25% of the time). All penetrations and aspirations were silent in nature with no changes in physiologic status or negative reactions.

Therapy included thickening liquids to a hot syrup consistency and giving them via standard nipple. With these interventions, Jamie demonstrated better fluid expression, increased control, and organization. He was able to take 10 cc in a matter of minutes without any difficulty. The amount of feeding that Jamie would take depended on the feeder. Some nurses were able to feed him up to 70 cc for three consecutive feedings. Others believed that he did not like thickened formula and would either not try or stopped feeding after 10 minutes. He continued to refuse feedings after 15 minutes, which may indicate a further decline in skills and subsequent aspiration. Jamie received a G-tube to improved weight gain. Oral feedings of thickened liquids were presented as tolerated and not forced.

Summary

This case illustrates how some infants may not show signs of aspiration during a feed when indeed they are aspirating. Diagnosing all of Jamie's medical conditions proved to be a lengthy process. This case also illustrates the importance of the videofluoroscopic swallow study as part of the diagnostic process and the need for cooperation among the different individuals involved in feeding an infant with dysphagia.

SECTION

GLOSSARY

· ·

A and B spells: apnea and bradycardia or "As & Bs." Apnea is a lack of breathing for longer than 15–20 seconds. Bradycardia is a slower than normal heart rate. A & B spells may occur during feeding and signal the feeder that the infant is not tolerating the feeding.

ABO incomp: incompatibility within ABO blood groups. ABO is a classification system of human blood types relative to their compatibility for transfusion. Blood types are A, B, AB, and O.

Abscess: a localized collection of pus that is usually the consequence of bacterial infection.

Achalasia: failure or incomplete opening of the lower esophagus sphincter. Achalasia can also occur at the upper esophageal segment (cricopharyngeal achalasia).

Acidosis (acidemia): an excess of acid in the body tissue and in the blood.

Acute upper airway obstruction: blockage of the upper airway, usually caused by aspiration of a foreign body. Results in respiratory insufficiency marked by progressive hypoxemia. The alveoli fill with fluid, which interferes with gas exchange. Sometimes referred to as acute respiratory distress syndrome (ARDS).

Adjusted chronologic age (ACA): the age a preterm infant would be if born at term; used in assessment of developmental milestones; same as corrected age.

Agenisis of the corpus callosum (ACC): congenital absence of the corpus callosum, a band of commissural fibers connecting the two cerebral hemispheres.

Alveoli: tiny sac-like spaces in the lungs. Oxygen and carbon dioxide are exchanged with the bloodstream across the alveolar lining.

Amblyopia: a loss of vision, centered in the brain, which develops over a period of time when the brain fails to receive proper signals from a weak eye.

Ampicillin: an antibiotic.

Anatomic dead space: any area of the air passages (nose, mouth, pharynx, larynx, trachea, bronchi, nonrespiratory bronchioles) containing air that does not participate in gas exchange (i.e., reach the alveoli during respiration). In a healthy infant, the volume of air in the anatomic dead space, measured in millimeters, typically is equivalent to the infant's weight in pounds.

Anemia: a reduction in the number of red blood cells circulating in the blood. It exists when hemoglobin content is less than that required to provide for demands of the body; common in premature infants.

Anencephaly: a congenital condition that is not compatible with life. The birth defect in which either the central nervous system (brain and spinal cord), or all but most primitive regions, are missing.

Ankyloglossia: a condition that occurs when the lingual frenulum, which connects the inferior surface of the anterior part of the tongue to the floor of the mouth, is short and interferes with tongue protrusion and elevation (a.k.a. tongue tie). The condition rarely interferes with nipple feeding, and surgical correction (frenotomy) is needed relatively infrequently.

Anomaly: a malformation of a part of the body.

Anoxia: a lack of sufficient oxygen.

Antibiotics: drugs that kill bacteria or interfere with their ability to grow and spread.

Antibodies: proteins produced by the body to fight harmful substances like viruses or bacteria that have entered the bloodstream.

Aorta: the artery leading from the heart that supplies oxygenated blood to the body.

Apgar score: a system for evaluating an infant's physical condition at birth based on a 0–10 scale. The infant's heart rate, respiration, muscle tone, response to stimuli, and color are rated at 1 and 5 minutes after birth.

Apnea: a lack of breathing for longer than 15–20 seconds; more severe spells may lead to bradycardia. **Central apnea** is caused by CNS problems and is characterized by no respiratory gas flow and no respiratory effort. **Obstructive apnea** is caused by an anatomic/physiologic problem and is characterized by continual respiratory effort but no respiratory gas flow. **Mixed apnea** is a combination of central and obstructive apnea.

Appropriate for gestational age (AGA): an infant whose size, weight, and growth is between the 10th and 90th percentiles for his or her gestational age at birth regardless whether the infant was born at term, preterm, or posterm.

Arterial blood gas (arterial stick): a sample of blood taken from an artery to measure its oxygen, carbon dioxide, and acid content.

Arterial catheter (indwelling arterial catheter): a thin plastic tube placed in an artery to withdraw blood for testing and to measure blood pressure.

Artery: any blood vessel leading away from the heart. Arteries carry oxygenated blood to the body tissues (with the exception of the pulmonary artery, which carries nonoxygenated blood to the lungs from the heart).

Asphyxia: condition caused by insufficient intake of oxygen. An Apgar score at birth of 5 or lower is indicative of asphyxia.

Aspiration: the penetration of secretions or food below the level of the true vocal folds. This can interfere with effective air exchange (and lead to asphyxiation) or cause pulmonary inflammation (aspiration pneumonia). Aspiration may occur before, during, or after swallowing.

Aspiration pneumonia: inflammation and possible infection of the lung and bronchi caused by aspiration of foreign material.

Atelectasis: a respiratory disorder characterized by the lungs remaining partially or totally unexpanded (i.e., collapsed) at birth, preventing the respiratory exchange of carbon dioxide and oxygen (ateles = incomplete, ektasis = expansion).

Atrial septal defect (ADS): a hole in the wall between the two upper chambers of the heart.

Audiometric testing: tests administered to determine hearing loss.

Automatic phasic bite release pattern: small, patterned up-and-down jaw movements in response to sensory stimulation to the biting surfaces of the gums; diminishes after 5 months of age

Bacteria: single-celled organisms that can cause infection and disease.

Bagging: pumping air and/or oxygen into the infant's lungs by manually compressing a bag attached to a mask that covers the infant's nose and mouth.

Belly breathing: a normal respiratory pattern in infants caused by the diaphragm contracting and pushing against the abdominal wall. It is considered abnormal in young children with poor trunk support. The location of movements for respiration is the abdomen, with rib case flaring. In cases of increased respiratory effort, sternal depression may also occur.

Bicarbonate: a substance that may be given to an infant to neutralize excess acid in the blood.

b.i.d: an abbreviation derived from a Latin term, meaning twice daily.

Bililights: used as part of phototherapy to treat jaundice. The fluorescent lights help break down the bilirubin so it can be excreted by the infant; the infant wears protective patches over the eyes.

Bilirubin: yellow-orange color of bile formed by the breakdown of hemogloblin in red blood cells. In most newborns, the liver systems are not completely mature and bilirubin accumulates in the blood and skin, resulting in jaundice.

Bilirubin encephalopathy: brain damage caused by increased levels of bilirubin.

Blood gases: a blood test that measures the concentration of oxygen (PO), carbon dioxide (PCO), and the acidity of the blood (pH); helps determine the amount of oxygen and ventilatory support needed.

Blood pressure: the pressure exerted by blood against the walls of the blood vessels. This pressure causes blood to flow through arteries. There are two numbers given during a reading of blood pressure. The first number (also called the top number) is the systolic pressure, which tells the pressure exerted when the heart contracts, sending blood to the body. The second number (lower number) is the diastolic pressure, which tells the pressure exerted between heartbeats.

Blood type: there are four blood types: A, B, AB, and O. Blood types are classified according to the absence or presence of certain proteins. Blood is also classified as Rh positive or Rh negative, by the absence or presence of the Rh factor.

Bradycardia ("brady"): a slower than normal heart rate (in an infant = below 100 beats/minute; normal heart rates are 120–160 beats/minute); often occurs with apnea. Bradycardia is relative to each individual infant's "normal" resting heart rate. For example, premature infants typically have higher heart rates

(160–180 beats/minute). During work, such as feeding, it is common to see the heart rate increase 10 beats/minute over the baseline value.

Brain bleed: hemorrhaging into some part of the brain.

Brain death: an absence of messages or electrical impulses from the brain.

Brain stem evoked response audiometry: a way of testing for hearing loss in infants, in which the baby's brainwaves are measured in response to various sounds.

Bronchial tubes: the tubes that lead from the windpipe (trachea) to the lungs.

Bronchioles: little tubes that branch off from the larger bronchial tube.

Bronchiolitis: an infection or inflammation of the bronchioles.

Bronchitis: an infection or inflammation of the bronchial tubes.

Bronchiectasis: irreversible dilation of the bronchial tree and destruction of the bronchial walls characterized by copious purulent sputum production. This condition may be congenital but is generally caused by previous inflammation or infection of the airway caused by aspiration of a foreign body.

Bronchodilator: a drug used to relax the contractions of the smooth muscles of the bronchioles to improve respiration.

Bronchopulmonary dysplasia (BPD) or chronic lung disease (CLD): a condition marked by respirator-induced (> 28 days) lung and bronchiole damage.

Bronchospasm: abnormal reflexive constriction of the airway in response to a variety of stimuli; often associated with a cough, wheezing, and mucus production. Can cause acute narrowing and/or airway obstruction.

Bubbling rale: abnormal respiratory sounds that indicate fluid movement in the lungs.

Buccal fat pads: also called sucking pads, are fat pads located in the cheek above the buccinator muscles. It is most prominent in young infants.

BUN (blood urea and nitrogen): a blood test that measures kidney and liver function.

Cachexia: general ill health, malnutrition, and emaciation associated with a serious disease such as cancer.

Café coronary syndrome: clinical syndrome of choking, facial cyanosis, and eventual collapse caused by acute upper airway obstruction; generally caused by aspiration of a bolus of meat.

Caffey's disease: also known as infantile cortical hyperostosis. This condition is characterized by swelling and tenderness of the affected area, particularly the mandible.

Caffey's syndrome: battered baby syndrome originally described by pediatrician John Caffey.

Calcium (Ca): a mineral element that aids skeletal development and contributes to the good health of the nervous, cardiovascular, and muscular systems.

Candida albicans (monila): a fungus known to cause yeast infections such as thrush.

Capillaries: very small blood vessels that remove waste from and provide oxygen and nutrients to body cells.

Carbon dioxide (CO_2): gaseous bodily waste product transported via the bloodstream and exhaled by the lungs.

Cardiology: medical discipline focusing on the heart and circulatory system.

Cardiopulmonary resuscitation (CPR): manual procedure for restarting or maintaining a person's breathing and heartbeat.

Catheter: thin tube used to drain or administer fluid.

Central line: an intravenous line threaded through a vein until it comes as close as possible to the heart.

Central nervous system (CNS): the spinal cord and brain.

Cerebral palsy (CP): an umbrella term for a group of nonprogressive, but often changing, motor impairment syndromes secondary to lesions or anomalies of the brain arising in the early stages of its development. Rarely occurs without associated defects such as mental retardation or epilepsy.

Cerebrospinal fluid (CSF): fluid that circulates around the spinal column and brain that has been produced by the ventricles of the brain.

CHARGE (coloboma, heart, atresia choanae, retardation, genitourinary, and ear): an association of multiple congenital anomalies. Children with CHARGE are usually neurodevelopmentally impaired, further complicating feeding issues. Tracheostomy appears to be the most effective means by which to manage the airway in these children.

CHD: abbreviation for congenital heart disease; also stands for congenital hip dislocation.

Cheek/lip retraction: abnormal pulling back of cheeks and lips for abnormal stabilization; seen with abnormal head and neck hyperextension and tongue retraction.

Chest tube: a tube placed in the chest cavity and connected to a suction system to remove trapped air or fluid, allowing lungs to expand.

Chewing: to break solid foods for swallowing through rotary jaw movements, lateral spreading of tongue, posterior transit with tongue, and buccal tension to hold food between teeth and cheeks.

Choanal atresia or stenosis: a lesion (either membranous or bony) in the nasal airway, resulting in a failure of the oronasal membrane to rupture (at about 6 weeks gestation). Patients with bilateral choanal atresia have cyclical periods of cyanosis at rest or at feedings, which are relieved when the child begins to cry and breath through its mouth, relieving the nasal airway obstruction. A return to the resting, noncrying state ensues and the cycle begins again. Bilateral choanal atresia makes it impossible for an infant to suck, swallow, and breathe in a coordinated way. Thus, oral feeding is usually impossible. Surgical repair to provide a patent nasal airway is usually completed in the neonatal period.

Chronic aspiration: repeated or intractable episodes of aspiration.

Chronic bronchitis: clinical syndrome of sputum production for at least 3 months in each of 2 successive years in a patient in whom other causes of chronic cough have been excluded.

Chronic obstructive pulmonary disease (COPD): a disease process that decreases the ability of the lungs to perform ventilation. Diagnostic criteria include a history of persistent dyspnea on exertion, with or without chronic cough, and less than half of normal predicted maximum breathing capacity. Diseases that cause this condition are chronic bronchitis, pulmonary emphysema, chronic asthma, and chronic bronchiolitis.

Chyme: the mixture of partly digested food and digestive secretions found in the stomach and small intestines during digestion of a meal. It is a varicolored, thick, nearly liquid mass.

Cleft lip: a congenital defect resulting from the faulty fusion of the median nasal process and the lateral maxillary processes; usually unilateral and on the left side, but may be bilateral.

Cleft palate: a congenital defect resulting from incomplete fusion of the horizontal palatal segments.

CLD: an abbreviation for chronic lung disease, also called bronchopulmonary dysplasia.

Compensation: lessening of a swallowing (or other) problem by learned behavior, increased use of alternative mechanisms, or the inherent plasticity of the nervous system and of swallowing functions. Compensation may occur through use of postures that change pharyngeal dimension and redirect bolus flow, through adaptations in bolus volume, bolus delivery or consistency, or through the use of sensory reinforcements or prostheses.

Complete blood count (CBC): a blood test done to determine the number of cells (red, white, and platelets) present in an infant's blood.

Computed tomography (CT): term referring to a specialized x-ray examination that produces thin (usually 10-mm thick) cross-sectional reconstruction of the body using computer back-projection techniques.

Controlled, sustained bite: graded closure of the teeth through food with equally graded release for chewing; seen at 11–12 months of age.

Corrected age: the age a premature infant would be if born on the due date.

CPAP (continuous positive airway pressure): pressurized air, sometimes with additional oxygen, that is delivered to the infant's lungs to keep them expanded as the infant breathes; maintains positive air pressure in airways throughout cycle, allowing patient to exhale against positive pressure.

Cricopharyngeal bar: posterior impingement of the pharyngoesophageal junction lumen as seen during radiographic studies. Symptomatic primarily in context of Zenker's diverticulum.

CSF: abbreviation for cerebrospinal fluid.

Cultures: tests performed as a part of a septic workup to look for bacteria, fungus, or a virus.

Cyanosis: a blue color of the skin caused by a lack of oxygen; reduced hemoglobin.

Cystic fibrosis: an inherited disease caused by mutation in a membrane chloride channel and characterized by excessive production of tenacious mucus and repeated respiratory infection. An autosomal dominant disorder that is the most common lethal genetic disease involving Caucasian children (approximately 1:2,000 live births).

Cytomegalovirus (CMV): a type of virus that may infect an unborn infant causing a severe illness, birth defects, and mental retardation. The virus can also infect an infant after birth. CMV also stands for continuous mandatory ventilation.

Decannulation: the removal of a tracheostomy tube.

Decerebrate posture: a sign of brain damage in which the upper extremities are extended and internally rotated, and the legs are extended with the feet in a forced plantar flexion.

Decorticate posture: a sign of brain damage in which the upper extremities are rigidly flexed at the elbows and wrists.

Deglutition: the act of swallowing, beginning with oral preparation of food and ending with esophageal transit of food into the stomach.

Dexamethasone: a steroid sometimes used following a brain injury, to help reduce swelling in the brain, that can be used to treat more severe chronic lung disease.

Dextrostix: (a) a blood test performed to assess sugar levels and (b) the plastic strip that has been chemically treated to be used for the test.

Diaphoresis: profuse sweating.

Diaphragmatic hernia: a congenital or traumatic protrusion of abdominal contents through the diaphragm.

Diffuse axonal injuries (DAI): widespead damage to nerve-cell axons throughout the brain caused by acceleration injuries (e.g., TBI).

Diffuse esophageal spasm: an esophageal motor abnormality characterized by the occurrence of simultaneous contractions during dry and wet swallows, which are predominantly seen in the smooth-muscle section of the esophagus. It commonly causes chest pain and dysphagia.

Dilantin (phenytoin): a drug that is often used to control seizures.

Direct therapy: therapy during which patients practice their swallow techniques with small amounts of food or liquid.

Disseminated intravascular coagulation (DIC): a condition in which the clotting factors and platelets in the blood are consumed due to infections, acidosis, hypoxia, or other injuries or diseases.

Diverticulum: a saccular deformation of an organ wall. In some diverticula, only the mucosal lining herniates through a dehiscence in the wall. In others, all layers of the wall form a permanent bulge. Diverticulae are named primarily for their sites: Zenker's diverticula form in the hypopharynx just above the upper esophageal segment. When large, undigested food may collect and putrefy in them. Midesophageal traction diverticula occur over the tracheal bifurcation; epinephric or pulsion diverticula occur in the distal esophagus.

Down syndrome: an abnormality in the chromosomes characterized by varying degrees of mental retardation and physical malformations.

DPT: abbreviation that refers to the immunizations against the diseases diphtheria, pertussis, and tetanus.

Ductus arteriosus: a blood vessel in the fetus that joins the aorta with the pulmonary artery in order to shift most of the blood away from the lungs. This blood vessel may not be closed in premature babies and must be closed by medicinal treatment or by surgery to enable proper blood flow and oxygen flow to the lungs.

Dysphagia: impaired swallowing; can occur anywhere from the mouth to the stomach.

Dysphagia lusoria: difficulty swallowing secondary to an aberrant right subclavian artery.

Dyspnea: air hunger resulting in a labored or difficult breathing, sometimes accompanied by pain.

Dystonia: prolonged muscle contractions that may cause twisting and repetitive movements or abnormal posture. These movements may be in the form of rhythmic jerks. The condition may progress in childhood, but progression is rare in adults. In children, the legs are usually affected first.

Echocardiogram: the graphic record produced by echocardiography.

Echocardiography: a noninvasive diagnostic method that uses ultrasound to visualize internal cardiac structures.

ECMO: abbreviation for extra corporeal membrane oxygenation.

Edema, edematous swelling: an accumulation of an excessive amount of fluid in cells, tissues, or serous cavities.

Electrocardiogram (ECG): a record of the electrical activity of the heart.

Electrodes: an apparatus attached to adhesive pads that are put on an infant's body to conduct electrical impulses of breathing motions and heartbeat to a monitor.

Electroencephalogram (EEG): the record obtained from an electroencephalograph.

Electroencephalography: amplification, recording, and analysis of the electrical activity of the brain.

Emesis: vomiting.

Empyema: pus in a body cavity, especially in the pleural space. It is usually the result of a primary infection in the lungs.

Endolarynx: structures within the laryngeal vestibule.

Endotracheal tube (ET tube): a thin plastic tube inserted into an infant's trachea to allow delivery of air/oxygen to the lungs through a respirator; see Section 7: Resources, "Feeding Equipment and Distributors."

Epilepsy: periodic convulsions or seizures caused by a disorder of the nervous system.

Eructate: to burp or belch

Esophageal atresia: congenital failure of the esophageal tube to develop.

Esophageal dilation: stretching of the walls of the esophagus to recover the lumen at the site of the strictures. Devices used for dilation include mercury-filled bougies, inflatable balloons, metal olives, and firm plastic rods of graded sizes.

Esophageal spasm: an abnormality characterized by the occurrence of simultaneous powerful contractions predominantly in the smooth muscle segment of the esophagus. Commonly causes chest pain and dysphagia.

Esophageal strictures: narrowing of the esophageal lumen, which leads to mechanical obstruction of the bolus passage. Strictures may be caused by webs, cancers (malignant strictures), or extrinsic compression (enlarged blood vessels, pulmonary tumors, goiters). Ingestion of lye may lead to formation of tight and tortuous fibrotic strictures. Peptic strictures are those occurring in reflux esophagitis; peptic strictures are short

and concentric. Treatment of strictures aims to recover the full size of the lumen, primarily through esophageal dilatation.

Esophagitis: inflammation of the esophagus, most commonly caused by gastroesophageal reflux, ingestion of corrosives, and infections. Mucosal lesions of typical esophagitis include erosions, exudate, or ulcerations that may lead to heartburn, chest pain, dysphagia, and odynophagia. Severe or chronic esophagitis may be complicated by formation of esophageal strictures or by mucosal metaplasia.

Esophagus: a tube that carries food from the mouth to the stomach.

Exaggerated jaw closure: excessive closure on feeding utensils to obtain external jaw stability during feeding to compensate for jaw instability.

Exaggerated tongue protrusion: excessive forward tongue movement with backward/forward movement of tongue similar to suckling pattern.

Exchange transfusion: blood transfusion in which the baby's blood is removed in small quantities while simultaneously being replaced with the same amounts of donor blood. Oftentimes, this is done to dilute harmful amounts of bilirubin.

Extremely low birth weight: infants weighing less than 800 grams.

Extubation: the removal of a tube from an organ, structure, or orifice, especially from the larynx after intubation.

Failure to thrive (FTT): a condition diagnosed in the first 2 years of life; a child's weight drops below the 3rd percentile of growth, with no known etiology.

Familial dysautonomia: hereditary disease common in Jewish cultures; characterized by dysphagia, absence of tears, indifference to pain, absent deep tendon reflexes, absent fungiform papillae on tongue, postural hypotension, emotional lability, excessive sweating, and abnormal esophageal motility.

Fine motor skills: skills involved in the coordination of small muscles such as those in the hand.

Fontanel: space between the unjoined sections of the baby's skull often referred to as the "soft spot."

Full term (FT): a term that describes a baby born at some point between the 37th and 42nd weeks of gestation.

Fundoplication: a surgical procedure in which the fundus (bottom-most part) of the stomach is wrapped around the distal esophagus. This procedure is recommended for older children (over 18 months of age) with life-threatening complications related directly to GER (choking, aspiration, recurrent apnea, chronic pulmonary disease, Barrett's esophagus, esophageal strictures, or large fixed hiatal hernias).

Gag response: a response to tactile input to the back of the tongue. It is very strong at birth, reducing in strength by about 7 months of age, and persisting through adulthood.

Gastroesophageal reflux: retrograde flow of gastric or biliary secretions from the stomach into the esophagus (and possibly the upper airway).

Gastroesophageal reflux disorder (GERD): chronic reflux of gastric contents into the esophagus, resulting in damage or symptoms.

Gastronomy: a surgically created opening in the abdominal wall to provide nutrition directly to the stomach; needed when the esophagus is blocked or injured, or to provide drainage after abdominal surgery.

Gastroschisis: a deficit in the abdominal wall resulting from a rupture of the amniotic membrane during physiological gut-loop herniation or later because of delayed umbilical ring closure, usually accompanied by protrusion of viscera.

Gavage feeding: forced feedings given through a tube passed through the nose or mouth and into the stomach.

Gentamicin: an antiobiotic.

Gestation: the length of time between the first day of the mother's last menstrual period before conception and the delivery of the infant.

Gestational age (GA): age computed from the first day of the last menstrual period to any point thereafter; usually not calculated beyond the first few months of life after birth.

Globus hystericus: a sensation as of a ball in the throat or as if the throat were compressed; a symptom of hysteria.

Glucose: the sugar that circulates in the bloodstream and is used by the body for energy.

Goiter: an increased size of the thyroid gland. Goiters are rarely of the size to cause mechanical obstruction of the bolus passage. However, thyroid disease is associated with various neuromuscular diseases, including myasthenia gravis.

Gram (G, GM, gm): the metric system's basic unit of weight; there are 28 grams in one ounce.

Gravida: a term used to specify pregnancy, a pregnant woman.

Guaiac test: a test for blood in the urine or feces using a reagent containing guaiacum, which yields a blue color when blood is present.

Haberman feeder: special feeder for infants with cleft palate; adjusts from fast to no flow.

Heart monitor: see Section 7: Resources, "Feeding Equipment and Distributors."

Heel stick: a method of taking small amounts of blood from an infant's heel for testing.

HELLP: an abbreviation for *h*aemophilus (bacteria found in the respiratory tract), *el*evated *l*iver enzymes, and *low p*latelets.

Hematocrit ("crit"): a measurement of the proportion of red blood cells in the blood.

Hemoglobin: iron-containing protein pigment occurring in the red blood cells of vertebrates and functioning primarily in the transportation of oxygen from the lungs to the tissues of the body.

Hemolysis: the rupturing of red blood cells.

Hernia: (a) umbilical—at the naval or umbilicus, a lump under the skin caused by a part of the intestine that protrudes through a fragile area of the abdominal wall; (b) inguinal—a lump under the skin in the groin area caused by part of the intestine protruding through a fragile part of the abdominal wall.

Hiatus hernia: protrusion of part of the stomach through the diaphragm into the thorax. This is an anatomical term and should not necessarily be equated with symptoms or a diseased state, although it is commonly associated with gastroesophageal reflux.

High risk: a term referring to people or situations needing special attention and intervention to ward off sickness (or keep it from worsening), damage, or death.

Human immunodeficiency virus 1 (HIV-1): a retrovirus that infects and destroys T cells, causing the marked reduction in their numbers that is diagnostic of AIDS (acquired immunodeficiency syndrome).

Huntington's disease: an inherited disease of the central nervous system characterized by progressive dementia and involuntary choreic movements, resulting from degeneration of the caudate and putamen nuclei; also called Huntington's chorea.

Hyaline membrane disease (HMD or RDS): see Respiratory distress syndrome.

Hydrocephalus: an abnormal accumulation of cerebrospinal fluid in the ventricles of the brain; can cause increased intracranial pressure and permanent brain damage and atrophy of the brain.

Hydrops fetalis: massive edema in the fetus or newborn, usually in association with severe erythroblastosis.

Hyperalimentation: IV fluid containing protein, vitamins, and minerals; used to provide nutrients to infants who cannot be fed milk.

Hyperbilirubinemia: excessive amount of bilirubin; commonly called jaundice; can cause liver damage.

Hypercalcuria: the presence of abnormally great amounts of calcium in the urine, resulting from conditions such as sarcoid, hyperparathyroidism, or types of arthritis with augmented bone absorption.

Hyperglycemia: excess of sugar in the blood.

Hyperkalemia: greater than normal amounts of potassium in the blood. This condition is seen frequently in acute renal failure. Early signs are nausea, diarrhea, and muscle weakness.

Hypermagnesemis: presence of excess magnesium in the blood serum.

Hypernatremia: (< 150) greater than normal concentration of sodium in the blood, caused by excessive loss of water and electrolytes resulting from polyuria, diarrhea, excessive sweating, or inadequate water intake.

Hypertension: abnormally high arterial blood pressure.

Hypertrophic pyloric stenosis: the only common malformation of the stomach. A marked thickening of the pylorus (distal sphincteric region of the stomach) is noted. Both the circular and longitudinal muscles in the pyloric region are hypertrophied. Severe narrowing of the pyloric canal results in obstruction of the passage of food. The infant presents with projectile vomiting.

Hyperventiliation: abnormally high breathing.

Hypocalcemia: Calcium levels in the blood that are too low.

Hypoglycemia: abnormal decrease in sugar in the blood.

Hypokalemia: (< 3) a condition in which an inadequate amount of potassium is found in the circulating bloodstream; characterized by abnormal ECG (electrocardiogram), weakness, and flaccid paralysis; may be caused by starvation, treatment of diabetic acidosis, adrenal tumor, or diuretic therapy.

Hyponatremia: a less than normal concentration of sodium in the blood caused by inadequate excretion of water or by excessive water in the circulating bloodstream. In a severe case, the person may develop water intoxication, characterized by confusion, lethargy, leading to possible muscle excitability, convulsions, and coma.

Hypopharyngeal diverticula: outpouching of the muscular pharyngeal wall above the cricopharyngeal muscle.

Hypoplasia: a condition of arrested development in which an organ or part remains below the normal size or in an immature state.

Hypotension: decreased cerebrospinal fluid or respiration failure; can result in coma or death.

Hypothermia: abnormally low blood pressure.

Hypotonia: abnormally low muscle tone.

Hypoxemia: insufficient oxygen in arterial blood.

Hypoxia: a lack of sufficient oxygen; deficiency of oxygen reaching tissues of the body.

Hypoxic encephalopathy: brain damage caused by hypoxia.

I and O: an abbrevation for input and output/outflow referring to the amount of fluids given and the amount of fluids excreted, as well as blood removed for testing over a period of time.

Ileostomy: an opening in the abdominal wall created by surgery to all the ileus (part of the intestine above the colon) to empty directly outside the body.

Ileus: obstruction of the bowel marked by painful distended abdomen, vomiting of dark or fecal material, toxemia, and dehydration.

Indirect therapy: exercise programs or swallows of saliva during which no food or liquid is given.

Indomethacin: a drug sometimes given to close the patent ductus arteriosus.

Infusion pump: a pump that delivers IV fluids in small, exactly measured amounts.

Intermittent mandatory ventilation (IMV): mode of cycled ventilation in which patient may breath spontaneously between timed mandatory breaths.

Intermittent positive pressure ventilation (IPPV): mode of ventilation; there is enforced inflation of the lungs by the intermittent application of an increase of pressure to a reservoir of air supplying the lungs.

Intracranial hemorrhage (ICH): bleeding affecting or involving the cranium and cranila structures.

Intralipids: a solution of fats given in an IV over several hours each day; commonly given with hyperalimentation when an infant cannot be fed milk.

Intravenous (IV): a small needle or tube inserted into a vein to allow fluids into the bloodstream.

Intrauterine growth retardation (IUGR): infant who is smaller than normal for gestational age at birth; caused by malnourishment from placental insufficiency.

Intraventricular hemorrhage (IVH): bleeding within the ventricles of the brain; grade I is least extensive and grade IV most extensive.

Intubation: the insertion of a tube into the trachea to allow air into the lungs.

Isolette: a brand of incubator; an enclosed, heated bed in which an infant is kept until she or he no longer needs help in maintaining temperature.

IUGR (intrauterine growth restriction): a term used to describe an infant who is small for gestational age.

Jaundice: a yellow tint to the skin and the white of the eyes caused by excessive bilirubin in the blood.

Jaw stabilization: internal jaw control with minimal up/down jaw movements; important for cup drinking. Begins by the infant biting a cup at 13–15 months to active use of jaw muscles at 2 years.

Jaw thrusting: strong depression of lower jaw; the jaw may become stuck in open position; reinforces abnormal head and neck hyperextension.

Jaw thrusting with protrusion: strong depression with forward pushing of lower jaw; occurs as compensatory jaw movement to obtain stability.

Kanamycin: an antiobiotic.

Karagener's syndrome: a subset of the immotile cilia syndrome, characterized by the triad of bronchiectasis, nasal polyps or sinusitis, and situs inversus totalis.

Kernicterus: damage suffered by the nervous system that is caused by extremely high levels of bilirubin.

Kilogram (kg): a metric unit of measurement. One kilogram is equal to 1000 grams or 2.2 pounds.

Kwashiorkor: severe malnutrition in infants and children characterized by failure to grow and develop and changes in the pigmentation of the skin and hair caused by a diet excessively high in carbohydrates and low in protein.

Lactose: the sugar found in milk.

Lanugo: the fine, white, downy hair that covers a fetus' body; some premature infants are still covered in lanugo at birth.

Large for gestational age (LGA): newborn infant who is above the 90th percentile in weight at birth for her or his gestational age.

Large motor skills: the skills, like crawling and walking, that include coordination of large muscle groups.

Laryngeal cleft: a cleft in the larynx that may present with a cough during feeding. Stridor may be present at rest or increased with feeds; an anatomic abnormality resulting from incomplete closure of the tracheoesophageal septum or cricoid cartilage or both in the sixth to seventh week of fetal life.

Laryngeal diversion procedures: also known as subglottic closures, designed to separate the lower respiratory tract from the upper digestive tract without affecting the glottic or supraglottic parts of the larynx.

Laryngeal suspension: the elevation of suspension of the larynx to a position under the tongue where it is removed from the bolus path to avoid aspiration during swallowing.

Laryngeal vestibule: the structures comprising the endolarynx, bounded by the rim of the epiglottis, superior edge of the aryepiglottic folds, tips of the arytenoid cartilages, and superior edge of the interarytenoid space.

Laryngomalacia: anatomical abnormality in which flaccid supraglottic structures prolapse into the airway, with inspiration leading to stridor and even failure to thrive.

Laryngoscope: a utensil used in intubation to see the vocal folds and guide the tube between them.

Laryngospasm: a spasmodic closure of the glottic aperature; an exaggeration of the laryngeal adductory response in response to an aversive stimulus.

Laryngotracheal separation: a type of subglottic closure where the trachea is brought to the skin as a tracheotomy but the proximal segment is left closed as a blind pouch.

Lasix: a diuretic drug.

Lead wires ("leads"): the wires that lead from a monitor to its electrodes.

Lecithin: one of the ingredients used in the making of surfactant.

Leigh's disease: subacute necrotizing brain disease, or death of brain cells.

Leukocyte (white blood cells): this type of blood cell helps to protect the body against bacteria and viruses.

Lingual nerve: one of the branches of the trigeminal nerve that innervates the anterior portion of the tongue and carries input of sensory fibers responding to taste, touch, and pressure.

Lip pursing: cheek and lip corners are slightly retracted for abnormal stability while central portions of lips are puckered.

Lissencephaly: agenesis of the cerebral gyri; results in a smooth brain; no convolutions on the cerebrum.

Low birth weight (LBW): infant's weight less than 2500 grams or 5½ pounds.

Lower esophageal sphincter (LES): specialized muscle that closes the gastroesophageal junction and prevents gastroesophageal reflux by its tonic contraction; relaxes in response to swallowing.

Lower respiratory tract infection (LRI): an infection that can attack the lungs, bronchial tubes, voice box (larynx), or windpipe (trachea).

Ludwig's angina: soft-tissue infection of the deep tissue of the floor of the mouth.

Lumbar puncture (spinal tap): a medical procedure where spinal fluid is extracted from the lower back by inserting a needle between the vertebrae.

Lymphangioma: tumor formed of dialated lymphatic vessels.

Lymphatics: the vessels found in most organs that collect lymph and return it to the bloodstream via the thoracic duct.

Magnetic resonance imaging (MRI): a noninvasive diagnostic scanning technique that allows visualization of the soft tissues of the body by imaging the signal produced by the protons of soft tissues after a magnetic field in which a patient is placed has been perturbed by a second magnetic pulse. Allows scanning and reconstruction much like a CT scanning but with nonionizing radiation.

Mandibular hypoplasia: underdevelopment of the mandible as seen in some children with craniofacial anomalies (e.g., Pierre Robin sequence, hemifacial microsomias, Treacher Collins).

Marasmus: condition of chronic undernourishment occurring especially in children and usually caused by a diet deficient in calories and proteins but sometimes by disease or parasitic infection.

Meconium (mec.): greenish-black material present in the fetal intestinal tract before birth and usually contained in the infant's first bowel movement in the first days after birth. If excreted in utero, it may cause respiratory distress in the infant.

Meconium aspiration: the inhaling of meconium-stained amniotic fluid by the infant; serious respiratory problems may result.

Meconium staining: refers to amniotic fluid stained with meconium; may indicate the fetus was in distress before birth.

Meningitis: an infection or swelling of the meninges, the membranes found around the spinal cord and brain.

Meningocele: a birth defect where the tissue that lines the spinal cord and brain (meninges) bulges through an opening in the spinal column or skull.

Mental retardation (MR): intellectual development that is limited. There are various degrees of mental retardation.

Metachromatic leukodystrophy: hereditary, degenerative disease of white matter caused by a deficiency of sulfatase A.

Microcephaly: small head; may be associated with premature fusion of skull bones; can restrict brain growth and cause mental retardation if untreated.

Micrognathia: mandibular hypoplasia.

Midface hypoplasia: underdevelopment of the midface as in Crouzon and Apert syndromes.

Milk scan: a radionuclide test for aspiration where small amounts of radionuclide are placed in milk and ingested by an infant; see Section 7: Resources, "Feeding Equipment and Distributors."

Minimal brain dsyfunction (MBD): a syndrome that, because of problems with the central nervous system, causes behavioral difficulties and/or learning problems.

Minute ventilation (Ve): expired volume per unit time per kilogram of body weight. Oral feeding results in an impairment of ventilation during continuous sucking. The subsequent recovery during intermittent sucking depends on postconceptual age. The recovery or increase may be a complex phenomenon that begins with respiratory inhibition caused by frequent sucking and swallowing, followed by an increase in Ve as arterial CO_2 rises and the frequency of sucking and swallowing decreases.

Monitor: a mechanical device that records heart rate, pulse, blood pressure, oxygen saturation, respiration, or other vital signs.

Munching: early chewing pattern in which rhythmical up/down jaw movements help to spread and flatten food; begins at 5 months or with introduction of solids.

Myasthenia gravis: an autoimmune disease characterized by muscle weakness and progressive fatigue. It is caused by a functional decrease in the amount of acetylcholine at the neuromuscular junction, causing failure in inducing normal muscle contraction.

Myelomeningocele: spinal bifida with a portion of spinal cord and membranes protruding.

Myopia: Nearsightedness.

Nasal CPAP: continuous positive airway pressure administered to an infant through nasal prongs.

Nasal prongs: see Section 7: Resources, "Feeding Equipment and Distributors."

Nasogastric tube (NG tube): a small, flexible tube inserted though the nose or mouth into the stomach; used to gavage-feed an infant.

NBIC/NBICU: abbreviations for Newborn Intensive Care and Newborn Intensive Care Unit. The unit in the hospital where premature or sick infants can be cared for and monitored.

Nebulizer: a machine that humidifies air and/or oxygen that is passed to the infant.

Necrotizing enterocolitis (NEC): a gangrene-like condition of the intestinal tract that causes death of intestinal/colon tissue; can cause an orally aversive reaction in premature babies.

Neonate: a term used to describe an infant during the first 30 days of life.

Neuroaxonal dystrophy: familial degenerative disease of the CNS characterized by widespread axonal swellings with upper motor neuron and lower motor neuron involvement, nystagmus, optic neuropathy, and blindness.

Nippling: another term to describe bottle feeding.

Nissen fundoplication: surgical procedure used to treat gastroesophageal reflux. The fundoplication involves wrapping of the fundus of the stomach around the gastroesophageal junction.

Nonnutritive sucking (NNS): sucking for reasons other than nutrition. Could be on toys, pacifiers, and so forth. NNS has been shown to stabilize the heart rate, increase digestion during tube feedings, allow respiration to continue uninterrupted, and increase growth rate in premature infants. NNS should be two sucks per second faster than nutritive sucking (NS). NNS is not a prerequisite to NS.

Nosocomial: hospital-acquired; term usually used to refer to infections.

Nosocomial pneumonias: pneumonias, chiefly caused by gram-negative organisms, acquired in the hospital, especially in association with endotracheal intubation and mechanical ventilation.

NPO: abbreviation for a Latin term that means "nothing by mouth" or stop feedings.

Nucleus ambiguus: one of the cranial motor nuclei of the brain stem with motor neurons that innervate laryngeal, pharyngeal, and esophageal muscles.

Nucleus of the tractus solitarius: one of the cranial sensory nuclei of the brain stem that receives sensory input from the oral, pharyngeal, and laryngeal regions. Some of the sensory input is involved with taste. Interneurons within discrete subdivisions of the nucleus serve multiple functions, including controlling blood pressure, respiratory rhythmicity, swallowing, and taste.

Nutritive sucking (NS): sucking on a bottle or breast nipple to maintain nutrition.

Obstructive lung disease: a syndrome in which airflow out of the lungs is impeded by narrowing of the small or medium-size airway due to spasm, inflammation, or scarring. Overinflation of the lung, prolongation of expiration, air hunger, dyspnea, and respiratory insufficiency may result.

Odynophagia: pain on swallowing.

Omphalocele: a congenital defect that allows the intestines to protrude through an opening in the abdominal wall.

Oral intake: intake of nutrition by mouth.

Oral preparatory stage: stage of swallowing in which the tongue gathers the food bolus and forms it into a centrally located globular mass ready to be propelled over the back of the tongue.

Oral secretions: the mixture of saliva and organisms residing in the mouth.

Oral stage of swallowing: the voluntary first stage of swallowing in which a bolus is formed and propelled toward the pharynx through repeated contractions of the tongue.

Oropharyngeal transit time: the time taken between the beginning of swallowing and the time when the bolus passes out of the oropharynx.

Osteopenia: a condition where the bones become frail and breakable from loss of minerals.

Oto-acoustic emission (OAE): used as a part of newborn infant hearing screening. Sounds that are measured in the outer ear canal that are produced by the normal outer hair cells in the cochlea. The presence of these sounds may indicate normal hearing acuity in the newborn.

Oxygen (O₂): the gas that is responsible and imperative for supporting life.

Oxygen saturation: the amount of oxygen present in the blood and available for exchange at the tissue level, typically measured in capillary blood flow by a pulse oximeter with external sensor. The levels are expressed as a percentage of 100. A normal infant has oxygen saturation above 95% in most conditions. Premature infants may be considered to have acceptable saturation levels above 90%. Below 90% some degree of hypoxia is indicated.

Oxygen saturation monitor: device to monitor oxygen saturation in blood; measurement of the percentage of oxygen combined with hemoglobin relative to the maximum amount of oxygen the hemoglobin can contain.

Oxyhood: a plastic box that fits over the infant's head to provide oxygen and moisture; see Section 7: Resources, "Feeding Equipment and Distributors."

Patent ductus arteriosus (PDA): a condition common in premature infants in which the ductus (the fetal blood vessel connecting the aorta and the pulmonary artery) fails to close after birth; common problem that may require drug or surgical treatment.

Pavulon: a drug used to yield temporary paralysis.

Penetration: entry of oropharyngeal contents into the larynx above the true vocal folds. Some authors define penetration as entry into the trachea. It is important for authors to define their use of the term.

Percutaneous endoscopic gastronomy (PEG): feeding tube placed directly into the stomach from the skin, utilizing an endoscope for guidance.

Periodic breathing: three or more episodes of apnea lasting 3 seconds or more occurring within a 20-second period.

Peristalsis: a coordinated propulsive contraction of the esophagus that occludes the esophageal lumen to propel the bolus through the esophagus and into the stomach. When the contraction follows a pharyngeal swallow and begins at the cricopharyngeal level, it is a primary peristalsis. If the contraction is stimulated by residual bolus that has been left behind, or by distension (e.g., from reflux), it is called secondary peristalsis.

pH: a symbol for hydrogen ion saturation. A low pH means the solution is acidic.

Phenobarbital: a drug used to control seizures.

Phototherapy: a method of treating jaundice by placing lights (bililights) over the infant's bed to break down bilirubin.

Pill esophagitis: inflammation caused by the corrosive effects of medications that become lodged in the esophagus.

Placenta abruptio: premature separation of the placenta from the wall of the uterus, usually accompanied by bleeding.

Placenta previa: placenta is abnormally positioned over the cervix; can result in bleeding during middle or late pregnancy; cesarian delivery of the infant is often necessary.

Plasma: the part of the blood (clear and liquid in consistency) that is left when the red blood cells have been taken out.

Platelets: the part of the blood responsible for clotting.

Pleura: paired layers of connective tissue covering the lung (visceral pleura) and lining the inner chest wall (parietal pleura). Between these two layers, a potential space (the pleural space) can become filled with fluid (pleural effusion) or pus (empyema).

Plexus: anatomical network of nerves, veins, or lymphatic vessels.

Plummer-Vinson syndrome: dysphagia, iron-deficiency anemia, upper esophageal inflammation with web formation, angular stomatitis, and atrophic gastritis. Predominantly affects females between the ages of 40 and 70.

Pneumogram: a test that records infant heart rate and breathing pattern on a graph for an extended period of time when the infant is asleep; helps identify infants at risk for sudden infant death syndrome.

Pneumomediastinum: the presence of air or gas in the mediastinal tissues; may result from bronchitis, acute asthma, pertussis, cystic fibrosis, or bronchial rupture from cough or trauma. A potential complication of positive pressure mechanical ventilation or of the Heimlich maneuver.

Pneumonia: an infection in the lungs.

Pneumothorax: a collection of air in the pleural space (between lung and chest wall). When air fills this space, the lung collapses. A chest tube is inserted into the pleural space and connected to a drainage bottle, which allows the air pocket to empty and the lungs to re-expand.

Polycythemia: an excess of red blood cells.

Polyhydramnios: excess amniotic fluid at delivery; may indicate a lack of intrauterine sucking and swallowing, as seen in tracheoesophageal fistula or congenital diaphragmatic hernia.

Polymyositis: inflammatory disease of skeletal muscle, characterized by weakness.

Polyposis: presence of several polyps.

Polyradiculoneuropathy (Guillian-Barre syndrome): lower motor neuron paresis with rapid, symmetrical onset.

Positive and expiratory pressure (PEEP): mechanical ventilation of a small amount (5–20 cm H_2O) that applies positive pressure at the end of each expiration to keep collapsed alveoli open.

Postconceptual age: the number of weeks following conception; approximately 2 weeks less than gestational age.

Postprandial reflux: reflux that follows eating a meal.

Postural strategies: changing of the patient's head or body posture (to eliminate aspiration), which changes the dimension of the pharynx and the direction of food flow without increasing the patient's work or effort during swallow.

Pre-eclampsia (toxemia): a complication of pregnancy that may cause protein in the urine, high blood pressure, rapid weight gain, and swelling from fluid retention in the mother. The disease can worsen into eclampsia, a life-threatening condition for mother and infant.

Premature rupture of the membranes (PROM): breaking of the amniotic membranes before the expected delivery date.

Prematurity: an infant who is born before 38 weeks gestation is premature. These infants may have underdeveloped lungs and require ventilation support. Anatomic structures are present, but they have decreased body fat, decreased postural control, underdeveloped fat pads (sucking pads), and underdeveloped sensorimotor systems. They may have difficulty coordinating suck, swallow, and breath. Extreme prematurity is less than 28 weeks. Because of technology, survival at 23 weeks is possible, but infants are not ready to feed orally until 31 weeks (breast) or 32 weeks (bottle) at the earliest.

Pseudomonas: a strain of bacteria.

Ptosis: drooping of the upper eyelid caused by injury to the ocularmotor nerve.

Pulmonary hypertension: the inability of the blood vessels in the lungs to relax and open following birth.

Pulmonary infiltrate with eosinophilia (PIE): hypersensitivity reaction, characterized by infiltration of alveoli with eosinophils and large mononuclear cells, edema, and inflammation of the lungs.

Pulmonary insufficiency of the premature (PIP): respiratory distress, caused by immature lungs and lack of surfactant, that attacks the youngest preterm infants.

Pulmonary interstitial emphysema (PIE): a situation created when bubbles of air are pushed out of the alveoli and in between the layers of lung tissue.

Pulse oximetry: a noninvasive method to determine arterial oxygen saturation using a probe placed on a highly oxygenated part of the body; see Section 7: Resources, "Feeding Equipment and Distributors."

Pyriform sinuses: spaces formed by attachment of the inferior pharyngeal constrictor muscles to the anterior portion of the thyroid cartilage. Food passes through the pyriform sinuses on the way to the esophagus.

Radiation absorbed dose (RAD): a unit of absorbed dose of ionizing radiation equal to 100 ergs per gram of absorbing material. This is a measure of the radiation dose a patient receives with x-rays or radionuclides.

Radiographic study/modified barium swallow: a diagnostic technique that uses barium and x-rays to view the oral and pharyngeal stages of swallowing.

RBC: abbreviation for red blood cells.

Real-time ultrasound: Ultrasound images that are reconstructed rapidly, allowing the operator to view the movement of the structures imaged at the same time the images are being taken.

Recurrent laryngeal nerve: a branch of the vagus nerve that provides partial sensory innervation to the larynx and motor innervation to the thyroarytenoid, lateral cricoarytenoid, interarytenoids, and posterior cricoarytenoid muscles.

Red blood cell (RBC, erthrocyte): the cells that carry oxygen and carbon dioxide to and from tissue.

Reflux esophagitis: inflammation of the esophageal mucosa, resulting from the reflux of gastric contents into the esophagus; a syndrome that can present clinically as heartburn, chest pain, or dysphagia.

Residual volume: The amount of air remaining in the lungs after maximal voluntary exhalation. This volume, which does not contribute to effective gas exchange, is increased in patients with obstructive lung diseases.

Residue: material left in the oral, pharyngeal, or laryngeal cavity after the swallow.

Respirator: see Section 7: Resources, "Feeding Equipment and Distributors."

Respiratory distress syndrome (RDS, CLD, HMD): Respiratory impairment found in premature babies whose bodies have not yet developed surfactant.

Retina: the nerve tissue that lines the back of the eye.

Retinopathy of prematurity (OP): abnormal growth of the blood vessels of the eye seen in many premature infants; this happens because the blood vessels are not finished developing at the time of a premature infant's birth. They have to finish developing outside the protected environment of the womb.

Retractions: indentations in the infant's chest during breathing; indicates difficulty breathing.

Room air: the air, containing 21% oxygen, that we normally breathe.

Rooting response: a reflex in which the infant turns its mouth toward tactile stimuli presented on the lips or cheeks. This reflex occurs at around 32 weeks gestational age and should disappear around 6 months of age.

ROP stage (right occipitoposterior presentation): the occiput of the fetus in relationship to the right sacroiliac joint of the mother in utero.

Rotary jaw movements: mature chewing pattern that involves up/down, forward/backward, lateral/diagonal, diagonal/rotary, and circular/rotary jaw movements.

Rx: abbreviation for prescription.

Santmyer swallow: a method to stimulate a swallow reflex by gently blowing a puff of air in the infant's face. This reflex is present in infants ranging from 33 weeks gestation to 11 months, but should be absent in neurologically normal children after the age of 2 years.

Scalp IV: an intravenous line placed in a baby's scalp vein.

Schatzki's ring (also known as B ring): a mucosal ring at the lower end of the esophagus, usually at the squamocolumnar junction. The upper surface of the ring is lined by squamous, esophageal epithelium, whereas the lower surface is lined by columnar gastric epithelium. It is typically seen in the setting of chronic gastroesophageal reflux and may be associated with a hiatal hernia.

Scintigraphy: images recorded by a gamma camera, which picks up the emissions of radionuclide energy from a patient after swallowing a radioactive substance. Allows for measurement of the amount of aspiration and residue in a patient.

Sepsis: a generalized infection that goes throughout the body through the bloodstream.

Septic workup: tests performed to check for infection.

Short-bowel syndrome (short-gut syndrome): malabsorption of nutrients induced after a massive small intestinal resection; some causes include necrotizing enterocolitis, midgut volvulus, multiple intestinal atresias, intestinal malrotation, and abdominal wall defects.

Shunt: an artificially created passage between two parts of the body used to drain excess fluid. A ventriculo-peritoneal shunt drains fluid from the ventricles of the brain into the peritoneum (abdominal cavity) for children with hydrocephalus.

Sialorrhea: production of excess saliva; drooling.

Sicca syndrome/Sjogren syndrome: dryness of the mucous membrane in head and neck; could cause the tongue to be sore, coated, and fissured. Sjogren syndrome refers to gland destruction by autoimmune disease, including rheumatoid arthritis and lupus. Gland destruction or malformation also occurs from radiation, excision, dehydration, and drugs.

Sleep apnea: a periodic cessation of breathing during sleep, often related to airway collapse from weakness of pharyngeal muscles. Symptoms include irregular breathing and loud snoring during sleep and excessive daytime sleepiness.

Small for gestational age (SGA): a newborn whose weight is lower than expected for gestational age.

Spillage: material that falls into the pharynx before the pharyngeal swallow response begins.

Sphingomyelin: an ingredient used in the making of surfactant.

Spinal tap (lumbar puncture): a medical procedure where spinal fluid is extracted from the lower back by inserting a needle between the vertebrae.

Squeeze pressure: pressure exerted on a sensor as the lumen is cleared of contents and obliterated. During peristalsis of the pharynx and the esophagus, squeeze pressures typically follow and exceed bolus pressures.

Stenosis: a narrowing or constriction.

Strabismus: a disorder of the eye muscles that may cause the eyes to cross (esotropia) or turn outward (exotropia).

Stridor: a noise heard during respiration indicating obstruction of the airway.

Subarachnoid hemorrhage: bleeding around the outer area of the brain (subarachnoid space).

Subglottic stenosis: a narrowing in the trachea below the level of the glottis that may result in airway obstruction.

Sucking: the act of drawing liquids into the oral cavity through negative pressure. Negative pressure is created by sealing the lips around the object and moving the tongue repeatedly up and down.

Suckling: a form of sucking present in the first few months of life in which forward and backward movements of the tongue help remove liquids from a nipple for feeding.

Suckling bursts: ratio of sucks to swallows. In a normally developing infant, this ration is 1–2 sucks per swallow.

Suction catheter: see Section 7: Resouces, "Feeding Equipment and Distributors."

Surfactant: a complex mixture of phospho-lipids (chiefly lecithin and sphingomyelin) secreted by alveolar type II cells that reduce the surface tension of the pulmonary alveoli in the lungs and thus reduce the tendency of the alveoli to collapse.

Swallow apnea: the normal interruption of the respiratory cycle during a swallow.

Synchronizer: see Section 7: Resources, "Feeding Equipment and Distributors."

Syringobulbia: cavities or holes in the medulla.

Tachycardia: an abnormally fast heart rate; in an infant, above 160 beats per minute.

Tachypnea: an abnormally fast breathing rate; in an infant, above 60 breaths per minute.

Temperature probe: see Section 7: Resources, "Feeding Equipment and Distributors."

Term infant: an infant born between the 38th and 42nd week of gestation.

Theophylline: a stimulant drug sometimes used in the treatment of apnea.

Thermoregulation: the regulating of body temperature.

Thoracic-abdominal breathing: a respiratory pattern characterized by expansion of the thoracic and upper abdominal areas on inhalation, in which the rib cage elevates and laterally expands while the diaphragm contracts and lowers. This causes vertical expansion and is evident as early as 7–8 months.

Thrombocytopenia: abnormal decrease in the number of platelets in blood.

Thrush: a fungal infection of the mouth.

Tongue lateralization: side-to-side movement of the tongue to maintain and move food to the teeth during chewing; begins at 6–7 months.

Tongue pumping: repeated front to back rocking-like motion of the tongue preceding swallowing.

Tongue retraction: pulling the tongue back for abnormal stability; reinforces abnormal head and neck hyperextension.

Tongue retraction with anterior tongue elevation: abnormal stabilization of tongue back in oral cavity with tongue tip elevated against hard palate; done to compensate for excessive tongue instability.

Tonic biting: abnormally strong jaw closure in response to touch on biting surfaces.

TORCH study: Tests for the following viral infections: toxoplasmosis, rubella, cytomegalovirus, herpes, and others (AIDS, syphillis, hepatitis).

Total parenteral nutrition (TPN): nutritional needs provided exclusively through intravenous access and not the gastrointestinal tract; also called a central line.

Toxic aspirations: inhalation of substances such as strong acids, strong bases, or petrochemicals, which can lead to rapid direct injury to the air spaces.

Trachea: the windpipe, which extends from the throat to the bronchial tubes.

Tracheal intubation: placement of a tube into the trachea to assist with breathing; placement is either translaryngeally or via a tracheostomy.

Tracheoesophageal fistula (TEF): an abnormal hole between the trachea and esophagus that allows a bolus to enter the trachea causing symptoms similar to aspiration.

Tracheoesophageal separation: a type of surgical intervention where the subglottic trachea is brought to the skin as a tracheotomy, but the supraglottic portion of the larynx is attached to the esophagus so all ingested food entering the larynx can exit into the esophagus.

Tracheotomy: a surgical procedure in which an incision is made between tracheal rings, below the level of the vocal folds, to help a person breathe.

Transcutaneous oxygen monitor (TCPO): continuously monitors an infant's blood oxygen level at the skin surface through a sensor placed on the infant's abdomen or chest; see Section 7: Resources, "Feeding Equipment and Distributors."

Transient lower esophageal sphincter relaxation (TLESR): relaxations of the lower esophageal sphincter that occur without associated swallowing activity. These events account for 60–80% of gastroesophageal reflux events.

Tubal feeding: feeding using a liquid formula passed into the enteral tract via tubes placed through either the mouth or nose.

Ultrafast computed tomography: synonymous with fast CT scanning. A technique of CT scanning in which the x-ray rapidly scans the patient in several planes; fast enough to freeze rapid motions such as the ones that occur in the oropharynx during swallowing.

Ultrafast MRI: a scanning technique using certain sequences of magnetic pulses allowing rapid magnetic resonance imaging scans to be performed.

Ultrasound imaging: a method of evaluating the soft tissues using high-frequency sound waves to create images. Tissue contrast is provided by the differences in each tissue's ability to reflect sound; see Section 7: Resources, "Feeding Equipment and Distributors."

Umbilical artery catheter (UAC): a tube placed into an artery in the umbilical cord to give medication and IV fluid or to draw blood; see Section 7: Resources, "Feeding Equipment and Distributors."

Unilateral: referring to only one side of the body.

Upper esophageal sphincter (UES): formed by the cricopharyngeus muscle, this is the top sphincter along the esophagus that is responsible for opening the esophagus to allow a bolus to enter and keeping material from flowing back up into the esophagus. Opening of the UES segment is enhanced by the pull from the hyoid ascent and the pressure exerted by the luminal bolus.

Upper GI study (UGI): a fluoroscopic study used to evaluate the anatomical structures in the esophagus, stomach, duodenum, gastric outlet, and proximal small bowel.

Upper respiratory infections (URI): an infection in the airways above the voice box (larynx).

UTI: abbreviation for urinary tract infection.

Vagus nerve: the 10th cranial nerve, which arises from the lateral side of the medulla oblongata and innervates a wide variety of visceral organs including the tongue (sensory), pharynx (sensory and motor), larynx (sensory and motor), and lungs and heart (parasympathetic and visceral afferent).

Valleculae: the space between the base of the tongue and the epiglottis. One point where a swallow can be triggered.

Valsalva maneuver: producing a forceful expiration against a closed glottis.

Vasovagal response: fainting.

Vasovagal syndrome: a paroxysmal condition marked by slow pulse and fall in blood pressure caused by stimulation of the vagus nerve, mediated through the carotid sinus.

Vein: a blood vessel that goes to the heart, carrying nonoxygenated blood.

Very low birth weight: infants weighing less than 1000 grams.

Ventricle: (a) a tiny chamber, as in those of the heart; (b) tiny chambers in the middle of the brain where cerebrospinal fluid is created.

VFE (videofluoroscopic examination): examination of oral and pharyngeal swallowing function using barium-coated food and liquid and x-ray equipment. Also called dysphagia diagnostic study (DDS), functional assessment of swallowing (FAS), videofluoroscopic swallow study (VFSS), cookie swallow test, and modified barium swallow (MBS). The primary purpose of this examination is to determine the cause(s) of dysfunction of the oral and/or pharyngeal stages.

Virus: a small infectious organism that thrives in the cells of the body.

Vital signs: pulse rate, rate of respiration, and body temperature.

Warmer: see Section 7: Resources, "Feeding Equipment and Distributors."

Waterbrash: a gush of saliva produced in response to reflux.

WBC: abbreviation for white blood cells.

Wilson's disease (Hepatolenticular degeneration): an hereditary disease in which decreased serum ceruloplasmin and copper cause copper deposits in the tissue and which is associated with cirrhosis, marginal pigmentation of the cornea, and CNS degeneration (basal ganglia).

Xerostomia: dry mouth caused by salivary gland dysfunction; can occur as a result of medication, disease, or radiation therapy.

Yeast: a miniscule fungus that can cause the occurrence of infections.

Zenker's diverticulum: herniation of the pharyngeal mucosa at the level of the upper esophageal sphincter. The diverticulum usually protrudes between the fibers of the cricopharyngeus and inferior constrictor muscles. These herniations most commonly occur on the left side, less commonly on the posterior wall and the midline, and only rarely on the right side.

Sources: Anderson, K., & Anderson, L. (1990). *Mosby's pocket dictionary of medicine, nursing, and allied health.* St. Louis, MO: C.V. Mosby. Batshaw, M., &

Perret, Y. (1998). *Children with disabilities: A medical primer* (4th ed.). Baltimore, MD: Paul H. Brookes. Harrison, H., & Kositsky, A. (1983). *The premature baby book.* New York: St. Martins Press. www.aapi-online.org/nicuglossary.htm

SECTION

RESOURCES

· ·

INTERNET SITES[1]

Syndromes and Disorders

Sites with information on cleft lip and palate, craniofacial syndromes, resources, and links to other craniofacial sites:

jamestgoodrich.com/craniofacial-syndromes.html

widesmiles.org/

cleft.com

Birth defects and syndromes with information given in both English and Spanish; includes links to other pertinent sites:

http://www.modimes.org/

---

[1] At the time of publication, the Internet sites listed here were available. Given the nature of the medium, however, there is no guarantee that these sites are still available or that they have not changed addresses.

Gastroesophageal reflux and other GI disorders:

http://www.aboutdigestion.com/script/main/art.asp?articlekey=375

www.pediatric-gi-center.com

www.hsc_virginia.edu/cmc/tutorials/reflux/references.htm

www.nationaljewish.org/medfacts/reflux.html

www.mednetslgerd.htm

www.sam.brooks.af.mil/web/af/afc/gastroesophageal%20Reflux%20disorder.htm

Breast feeding for children with feeding issues:

http://wwwwidesmiles.org/cleftlinks/feeding.html

www.inxpress.net/~paisans/CF/Feed.html

General references on many pediatric diseases:

http://www.medline.net/symptoms/diff_swall.htm

http://www.icondata.com/health/pedbase/files/ACUTEUVU.htm

http:// www.neurosurgery.medsch.uc la.edu/Diagnoses/Pediatric/PediatricDis_Intro.html

http://www.neonatology.org/syllabus/syllabus.html

http://medlib.med.utah.edu/WebPath/PEDHTML/PEDIDX.html

http://neurosurgery_mgh.harvard.edu:80/pedi-hp.htm

http://www.dysphagia.com/diseases.htm

http://www.mic.ki.se/Diseases/index.html

http://www.familyvillage.wisc.edu/education/ei.html

http://www.csun.edu/~hcmth011/heart/

http:// medwebplus.com/ subject/ Pediatrics/Diseases_and_Conditions.ht ml

Down syndrome:

http://www.modimes.org/HealthLibrary2/factsheets/Down_Syndrome.htm

www.ds-health.com/ds_sites.htm

Upper airway problems in children:

http://www.vh.org/Providers/Textbooks/ElectricAirway/ElectricAirway.html

www.gretmar.com/webdoctor/entped.html

Prader-Willi syndrome:

http://www.icondata.com/health/pedbase/files/PRAOER-W.HTM

Embryology

www.med.uc.edu/embryology

www.screamer.bsd.uchicago.edu/sections/neurosurg/neuroreview/01-embryology/index.html

www.calluso.med.mon.ca/~tscott/embryo/emb.htm

www.barteby.net/107/3.html

www.newcastle.edu.au/department/md/anatomy/bmd1_20/mr2_int.htm

www.home.stny.rr.com/science/biology/embryology.html

www.neonatology.org/

www.ama-assn.org

www.sciam.com/1999/0399issue/0399smith.html

www.visembryo.com.

Premature Birth

www.kennedykrieger.org/familyreso/services/feeding.html

www.jazz.san.uc.edu/~pranikjd/premie.html

www.bflrc.com/newman/overheads/prematures.htm

www.babyparenting.miningco.com/msubpreem.htm

www.parentandchild.com/articles/1166.html

www.comeunity.com/premature/index.html

www.mondenet.com/~chrisck/preemies.htm

www.comeunity.com/premature/child/growth/index.html

Feeding

www.neonatology.org/syllabus/feeding.premature.html

http://www.hcn.net.au/healthbrochures/feeding/intro.htm

http://home.earthlink.net/~leedlelop/anne4.htm

http://www.unmc.edu/Community/npp/feed34.htm

http://www.cyberparent.com/bfed2/

http://www.carnationbaby.com/Y/Ya2a.html

http://www.health.gov.ab.ca/public/nutrit/feedbaby.htm

http://www.ama-assn.org/insight/h_focus/nemours/baby/feeding/newborn.htm

http://www.nncc.org/Nutrition/feed.infants.html

http://www.health-net.com/breast.htm

http://www.babybag.com/articles/babyfood.htm

http://www.state.sd.us/doh/Pubs2/infant.ht

http://www.zerotothree.com

http://www.bestfed.com

http://www.kidshealth.org/parent/growth/feeding/feednewborn_p2.html

http://www.babiesonline.com

http://www.dysphagia.com/dx.htm

http://dyspahgia.com/asha_SID_13.htm

www.appstate.edu/~clarkhm/pediatric/adultped.htm

www.nmmc.com/nmhc/services/rehab/swallow.htm

www.dysphagia-diet.com/index.htm

www.dysphagia.com/diseases.htm   www.chop/clinical/seashorehouse/html/dysphagia.html

Diagnostic and Assessment Procedures

Upper GI series in infants barium swallow:

http://drad.umn.edu/pedrad/teach/cvhtml/002/ca002.htm

http://salon.drkoop.com/adam/peds/top/003816.htm

Diagnosis of Esophageal Disorders

http://salon.drkoop.com/adam/peds/top/003401.htm

http://salon.drkoop.com/adam/peds/top/003884.htm

http://www.bgsm.edu/voice/pediaticreflux.html

http://kidshealth.org/ai/service/generalpedsurgery.reflux.html

www.childrens-seashore.org/htm/dysphagia.htlm

www.appstate.edu/~clarkhm/pediatric/pedout5.htm

Management Services

www.doctorindex.com/topics/dysphagia.html

www.slackinc.com/child/pednet-p.htm

Cookbooks and Other Products for Feeding Therapy

www.thickandeasy.com/aip-swalnew.html

www.singpub.com/product/0396.html

www.fnms.com/dysphagi.htm

www.preemies.com

www.feeding.com

General Health and Medical

www.health-net.com

www.health-library.com/

www.zorcom.com/general_health.htm

www.intelihealth.com/IH/IHTIH/WSIHWOOO/333/341/273239.html

www.familyinternet.com/navigate_menu/sites/family_health.html

www.100tophealthsites.com

www.family.go.com/categories/parenting

www.bewell.com

http://www.disabilitynetwork.com/

http://www.mchc.net/

Search Engines

www.yahoo.com

www.altavista.com

www.askjeeves.com

www.northernlight.com

www.mamma.com

www.search.aol.com

www.excite.com

www.alltheweb.com

www.looksmart.com

www.lycos.com

www.webcrawler.com

www.directhit.com

RESOURCES FOR CAREGIVERS OF CHILDREN WITH SPECIAL NEEDS

AIDS

National AIDS Hotline 1-800-342-AIDS (1-800-342-2437); 1-800-344-SIDA (1-800-344-7232 Spanish access); 1-800-AIDS-TTY (1-800-243-7889 Deaf access)

National AIDS Information Clearinghouse, PO Box 6003, Rockville, MD 20850 (1-800-458-5231; TTY/TDD: 1-800-243-7012)

Alcohol and Drugs of Abuse

Cocaine Babies: Florida's Substance-Exposed Youth (Available from Florida Department of Education, Prevention Center, Suite 414, FEC, 325 W. Gaines Street, Tallahassee, FL 32399)

AUTISM

Autism Society of America, 8601 Georgia Avenue., Suite 503, Silver Spring, MD 20910 (301-565-0433; FAX: 301-565-0834)

National Autism Hotline/Autism Services Center, Prichard Building, 605 9th Street, PO Box 507, Huntington, WV 25701-0507 (304-525-8014)

Breast Feeding

Lact-Aid International and Lact-Aid Moms Network, Box 1066, Athens, TN 37303 (800-228-1933; 615-744-9090)

Lactation Associates, 254 Conant Road, Weston, MA 02193-1756 (617-893-3553)

La Leche League International (LLL), PO Box 1209, Franklin Park, IL (601-31-8209; 312-455-7730)

Cerebral Palsy

United Cerebral Palsy Association, 7 Penn Plaza, Suite 804, New York, NY 10001 (1-800-USA-IUCP; 212-268-6655)

National United Cerebral Palsy Association, 1660 L Street Northwest, Suite 700, Washington DC 20036 (1-800-872-5827)

Cleft Lip and Palate

Cleft Palate Foundation, 104 South Estes Drive, Suite 204, Chapel Hill, NC 27514. Grandview Avenue, Pittsburgh, PA 15211 (919-933-9044; 800-24-CLEFT)

Cystic Fibrosis

Cystic Fibrosis Foundation, 6931 Arlington Road., Bethesda, MD 20814 (301-951-4422; 800-FIGHT CF or 800-344-4823)

Down Syndrome

National Down Syndrome Congress, 7000 Peachtree-Dunwoody Road, Building 5, Suite 100, Atlanta, GA 30328-1662 (800-232-6372)

National Down Syndrome Society, 666 Broadway, Suite 810, New York, NY 10012 (800-221-4602; 212-460-9330)

Epilepsy

Epilepsy Foundation of America, 4351 Garden City Drive, Suite 406, Landover, MD 20785 (301-459-3700; Information and Referral: 800-332-1000).

General

Clearinghouse on Disability Information, Office of Special Education and Rehabilitative Services, U.S. Department of Education, Room 3132, Switzer Building, Washington, DC 20202-2524 (202-732-1245; 202-732-1723).

March of Dimes Birth Defects Foundation, 1275 Mamaroneck Avenue, White Plains, NY 10605 (914-428-7100; 1-888-MODIMES [663-4637]; http://www.modimes.org/)

National Easter Seal Society, 230 West Monroe Street, Suite 1800, Chicago, IL 60606-4802 (312-726-6200; Toll free: 800-221-6827; http: //www.easter-seals.org). E-mail: esw@seals.org

Easter Seals Washington, 521 2nd Avenue West, Seattle, WA 98119 (800-678-5708; http://esw@seals.com)

National Organization for Rare Disorders, Inc. (NORD), PO Box 8923, New Fairfield, CT 06812 (203-746-6518; 800-999-6673; http:// www.rarediseases.org)

The National Tay-Sachs and Allied Diseases Association, 2001 Beacon Street, Suite 304, Brookline, MA, 02146 (617-277-4463; http://www.ntsad.org)

National Information Center for Children and Youth with Handicaps (NICHCY), PO Box 1492, Washington, DC 20013 (800-999-5599 or 703-893-6061)

National Sudden Infant Death Syndrome Foundation, Two Metro Plaza, Suite 205, 8240 Professional Place, Landover, MD 20785 (301-459-3388)

SKIP (Sick Kids Need Involved People), 216 Newport Drive, Severna Park, MD 21146 (301-647-0164)

Hearing, Speech, and Language

American Society for Deaf Children, 814 Thayer Avenue, Silver Spring, MD 20910 (301-585-5400; TDD: 301-585-5401)

American Speech-Language-Hearing Association, 10801 Rockville Pike, Rockville MD 20852 (301-897-5700 [Voice/TDD]; http:// www.asha.org)

Hydrocephalus

Hydrocephalus Foundation of Northern California, 2040 Polk Street, Box 342, San Francisco, CA 94109 (415-776-4713)

Mental Retardation

American Association on Mental Retardation, 444 North Capital Street NW, Suite 846, Washington, DC 20001 (202-387-1968; 1-800-424-3688; www.aamr.org)

Parents

Compassionate Friends, PO Box 1347, Oak Brook, IL 60522-3696 (708-990-0010)

The Exceptional Parent, 555 Kinderkamack Road, Oradell, NJ 07649 (800-372-7368)

Project COPE, 9160 Monte Vista Avenue, Montclair, CA 91763 (714-985-3116)

Spina Bifida

Spina Bifida Association of America, 4590 MacArthur Boulevard NW, Suite 250 Washington, DC 20007-4226. (Voice: 800-621-3141or 202- 944-3285; FAX: 202-944-3295; http://www.sbaa.org)

Syndromes

The 5p-Society (Cri du chat syndrome), 11609 Oakmont, Overland Park, KS 66210 (913-469-8900)

Educational material, including a newsletter, as well as referral sources are available for families.

International Rett Syndrome Association, Inc., 8511 Rose Marie Drive, Ft. Washington, MD 20744 (301-248-7031)

Educational materials for families, as well as referral sources, are available.

National Fragile X Foundation, 1441 York Street, Suite 215, Denver, CO 80206 (800-688-8765; 303-333-6155)

Educational materials for families, as well as referral sources, are available.

The National Neurofibromatosis Foundation, Inc., 141 5th Avenue, 7th Floor, Room 75, New York, NY 10010 (212-460-8980)

Educational materials for families and health professionals; offers genetic counseling and support groups.

Prader-Willi Syndrome Association, 6490 Excelsior Boulevard, Suite E-102, St. Louis Park, MN 55426 (612-926-1947)

This clearinghouse is a resource for information on Prader-Willi syndrome.

Support Organization for Trismoy 18, 13, and Related Disorders, c/o Barb Van Herreweghe, 2982 S. Union Street, Rochester, NY 14624 (716-594-4621)

Supplies resources and educational material to families with children with Trisomy 18 and Trisomy 13.

Traumatic Brain Injury

National Head Injury Foundation, Inc., 1140 Connecticut Avenue, NW, Suite 812, Washington, DC 20036-4002 (800-444-6443; 202-296-6443)

Educational materials and resources for individuals with traumatic brain injury and their families.

Vision

American Foundation for the Blind, Inc., 15 W. 16th Street, New York, NY 10011 (212-620-2020800/AFBLIND)

Blind Children's Center, 4120 Marathon, Los Angeles, CA 90029-0159 (1-800-222-3566)

FEEDING EQUIPMENT AND DISTRIBUTORS

The following distributor information is based on current information. Other distributors for the listed equipment may be available.

Equipment

NUK MASSAGE BRUSH

Smith Nephew Rolyan Inc.

PDP Products

Gerber Products Co.

New Visions

Equipment Shops

Local retail stores/pharmacies

SPOONS

❖ Maroon Spoons

Therapy Skill Builders

Equipment Shops

New Visions

PDP Products

❖ Rolyan Care Spoons

Smith Nephew Rolyan

FLEXI-CUT CUPS

Therapy Skill Builders

New Visions

PDP Products

Smith Nephew Rolyan

Equipment Shops

THERA-BAND TUBING

Smith Nephew Rolyan Inc.

PDP Products

Southpaw Enterprises Inc.

MAG MAG TRAINING CUP SYSTEM

Marshall Baby Products (contact for local retailers)
300 Lakeview Parkway
Vernon Hills, IL 60061
Equipment Shops

GERBER "GROW WITH ME" TRAING CUP SEt

Gerber Products Co.

New Visions

Local retail stores

IINFA-DENT (FINGER TOOTHBRUSH)

NU-TEC Health Products

New Visions

TY-D-SADDLE

Ty-D-Saddle
11810 Lake Hazel Road
Boise, ID 83709

New Visions (Sit Right Saddle)

MINI-MASSAGER BY HITACHI

Smith Nephew Rolyan Inc.

Southpaw Enterprises

THICK-IT

Milani Foods Inc.
2525 Armitage Avenue
Melrose Park, IL 60160

Bruce Medical Supply

MAMA CHAIR

MAMA Systems Inc.
4347 Silver Lake Road
Oconomowoc, WI 53066
414-567-8381

HABERMAN FEEDER

Medela Inc.
PO Box 660
McHenry, IL 60051-0660
800-435-8316

New Visions

Distributors

1. Therapy Skill Builders
   3830 E. Bellevue
   PO Box 42050-TS4
   Tucson, AZ
   602-323-7500

2. New Visions
   Route 1, Box 175-S
   Faber, VA 22938
   804-361-2285

3. Smith Nephew Rolyan, Inc.
   One Quality Drive
   PO Box 578
   Germantown, WI 53022
   800-558-8633

4. PDP Products
   12015 N. July Avenue
   Hugo, MN 55038
   612-439-8865

5. Equipment Shops
   PO Box 33
   Bedford, MA 01730
   617-275-7681

6. Gerber Products Company
   728 Booster Blvd.
   Reedsburg, WI
   800-4-GERBER

7. NU-TEC Health Products
   390 Oak Avenue, Suite A
   Carlsbad, CA 92008
   800-868-8338

8. Southpaw Enterprises, Inc.
   109 Webb Street
   Dayton, OH 45403-1144
   800-228-1698

9. Bruce Medical Supply
   411 Waverly Oaks Road
   PO Box 9166
   Waltham, MA 02254-9166
   800-225-8446

SECTION

REFERENCES

· ·

Agnagnostaki, D. (1980). Noise pollution in neonatal units: A potential health hazard. *Acta Paediatrica Scandanavica, 69,* 771–773.

Alexander, R. (1987). Oral-motor treatment for infants and young children with cerebral palsy. *Seminars in Speech and Language, 8,* 87–100.

Alexander, R., Arvedson, J., Dorsey, L., & Pinder, G. (1999, November). *Dysphagia and cerebral palsy through the life span.* Presentation at the American Speech Language Hearing Association, San Francisco, CA.

Alper, B., & Manno, C. (1996). Dysphagia in infants and children with oral-motor deficits: Assessment and management. *Seminars in Speech and Language, 17,* 283–310.

Als, H. (1982). Toward a synactive theory of development: Promise for the assessment and support of infant individuality. *Infant Mental Health Journal, 3,* 229–243.

Als, H. (1986). A synactive model of neonatal behavioral organization: Framework for assessment and support of the neurobehavioral development in the premature infant and his parents in the environment of the neonatal intensive care unit. In J. K. Sweeney (Ed.), The high-risk neonate: Developmental therapy perspectives, excerpted in *Physical & Occupational Therapy in Pedicatrics, 6,* 3–55.

Als, H., & Brazelton, T. B. (1981). A new model of assessing the behavioral organization in preterm and fullterm infants: Two case studies. *Journal of the American Academy of Child & Adolescent Psychiatry 1981 Spring, 20(2),* 239–63.

Als, H., Duffy, F., & McAnulty, G. (1988). Behavioral differences between preterm and fullterm newborns as measured with the A.P.I.B. system scores: I. *Infant Behavior & Development, 11,* 305–318.

Als, H., & Gilkerson, L. (1995). Developmentally supportive care in the neonatal intensive care unit. *Zero to Three, 15,* 1–10.

Als, H., Lawhon, G., Brown, E., Gibes, R., Duffy, F., Mcaunulty, G., & Glickman, J.

(1986). Individualized behavioral and environmental care for the VLBW preterm infant at high risk for bronchopulmonary dysplasia: NICU and developmental outcome. *Pediatrics, 78,* 1123–1132.

American Academy of Pediatrics, Committee on Environmental Health. (1997). Noise: A hazard for the fetus and newborn. *Pediatrics, 100,* 724–727.

American Gastroenterologic Association. (1994). An American Gastroenterologic Association medical position statement on the clinical use of esophageal manometry. *Gastroenterology, 107,* 865.

American Speech-Language-Hearing Association (2000). Skills needed by speech-language-pathologists providing services to dysphagic patients/clients. *ASHA, 32*(Suppl. 2), 7–12.

Anderson, K., & Anderson, L. (1990). *Mosby's pocket dictionary of medicine, nursing, and allied health.* St. Louis, MO: CV Mosby Company.

Arvedson, J. (1998). Management of pediatric dysphagia. *Otolaryngologic Clinics of North America, 31,* 453–476.

Arvedson, J., & Brodsky, L. (1993). *Pediatric swallowing and feeding: Assessment and management.* San Diego: Singular Publishing Group.

Arvedson, J., Rogers, B., & Brodsky, L. (1993). Anatomy, embryology, and physiology. In J. Arvedson & L. Brodsky (Eds), *Pediatric swallowing and feeding: Assessment and management* (pp. 5–52). San Diego: Singular Publishing Group.

Atkins, D., Lundy, M., & Pumariega, A. (1994). A multimodal approach to functional dysphagia. *Journal of the American Academy of Child & Adolescent Psychiatry, 33,* 1012–1016.

Babbitt, R., Hoch, T., & Coe, D. (1994). Behavioral feeding disorders. In D. Tuchman & R. Walter (Eds.), *Disorders of feeding and swallowing in infants and children: Pathophysiology, diagnosis, and treatment* (pp. 77–96). San Diego, CA: Singular Publishing Group.

BandenBerg, K. (1990). Nippling management of the sick neonate in the NICU: The disorganized feeder. *Neonatal Network, 9,* 9–16.

Barnard, K. I., Hammon, M., & Booth, C. (1989). Measurement and meaning of par-ent child interaction. In F. Morrisson, C. Lord, & D. Keating (Eds.), *Applied developmental psychology.* New York: Academic Press.

Bastian, R. (1998). Contemporary diagnosis of the dysphagic patient. *Otolaryngologic Clinics of North America, 31,* 489–506.

Batshaw, M. L., & Perret, Y. M. (1998). *Children with disabilities* (4th ed.). Baltimore, MD: Paul H. Brookes Publishing Company.

Battaglia, X., & Lubchenco, X. (1967). A practical classification of newborn infants by weight and gestational age. *Journal of Pediatrics, 2,* 159–63.

Beecher, R. (1994, October). *Pediatric swallowing and feeding disorders: Use of the oral pharyngeal motility study in assessment and management.* Inservice training for Advances in Continuing Education Programs-Pediatric Series. Detroit, MI: Henry Ford Hospital.

Bergstrom, L., & Owens, O. (1984). Posterior choanal atresia: A syndromal disorder. *Laryngoscope, 94,* 1273.

Berk, J. (1995). *Bockus gastroenterology.* Philadelphia, PA: W.B. Saunders Company.

Bernbaum J., Pereira, G., Watkins, J., & Peckham, G. (1983). Non-nutritive sucking during gavage feeding enhances growth and maturation in premature infants. *Pediatrics, 71,* 41–45.

Berry, M., Abrahamowicz, M., & Usher, R. (1997). Factors associated with growth of extremely premature infants during initial hospitalization. *Pediatrics, 100,* 640–646.

Blackburn, S. (1992). Alterations of the respiratory system in the neonate: Implications for the clinical practice. *Journal of Perinatal Neonatal Nursing, 6,* 461–464.

Blackman, J., & Nelson, C. (1985). Reinstituting oral feedings in children fed by gastrostomy tube. *Clincal Pediatrics, 24,* 434–438.

Blennow, G., Svenningsen M., & Almquist, B. (1974). Noise levels in infant incubators (adverse effects?). *Pediatrics, 53,* 29.

Boeckling, A. (1992). Exogenous surfactant therapy for premature infants. *Journal of Perinatal Neonatal Nursing, 6,* 59–66.

Bosma, J. (1967). *Symposium on oral sensation and perception.* Springfield, IL: Charles C. Thomas.

Bosma, J. (1985). Postnatal ontogeny of performances of the pharynx, larynx, and mouth. *American Review of Respiratory Disorders, 131,* 10–15.

Bosma, J. (1990) Evaluation and therapy of impairments of suckle and transitional feeding. *Journal of Neurologic Rehabilitation, 4,* 79–84.

Boyle, J. (1989). Gastroesophageal reflux in the pediatric patient. *Gastroenterology Clinics of North America, 18,* 315–337.

Brazelton, T. (1984). *The neonatal behavioral assessment scale. Second Edition. Clinics in Developmental Medicine. No. 88.* Philadelphia: J.B. Lippincott.

Brookshire, R. H. (1997). *Introduction to neurogenic communication disorders.* St. Louis, MO: Mosby.

Brown, L., & Hermann, J. (1997). The effect of developmental care on preterm infant outcome. *Applied Nursing Research, 10,* 190–197.

Bu'Lock, F., Woolridge, M., & Baum, J. (1990). Development of co-ordination of sucking, swallowing and breathing: Ultrasound study of term and preterm infants. *Developmental Medicine and Child Neurology, 32,* 669–678.

Canal, D., Vane, D., Gotto, S., Gardner, G., & Grosfeld, J. (1987). Changes in lower esophageal sphincter pressure (LES) after Stamm gastrostomy. *Journal of Surgical Research, 42,* 570–574.

Chatoor, I., Schaefer, X., Dickson, L., & Egan, J. (1984). Non-organic failure to thrive: A developmental prospective. *Pediatric Annals, 13,* 829–843.

Clark, J. (1993). Anatomy and physiology of the esophagus. In R. Wylie & J. S. Hyams (Eds.), *Pediatric gastrointestinal disease, pathophysiology, diagnosis and management* (pp. 311–317). Philadelphia: W. B. Saunders Company.

Committee on Pediatric AIDS. (2000). Identification and care of HIV-exposed and HIV-infected infants, children, and adolescents in foster care. *American Academy of Pediatrics. Committee on Pediatric AIDS. Pediatrics. 2000, 106,* 149–153.

Crelin, E. (1973). *Functional anatomy of the newborn.* New Haven, NJ: Yale University Press.

Crelin, E. (1987). *The human vocal tract.* New York: Vantage Press.

Curtis, J., & Langmore, S. (1997). Respiratory function and complication related to deglutition. In A. Perlman & K. Schulze-Delrieu (Eds.), *Deglutition and its disorders: Anatomy, physiology, clinical diagnosis, and management.* San Diego: Singular Publishing Group.

David, R. B., Gomez, M. R., & Okazaki, H. (1970). Necrotizing encephalomyelopathy (Leigh). *Developmental Medicine and Child Neurology, 12,* 436–445.

Davis, L. F. (1987). Respiration and phonation in cerebral palsy: A developmental model. *Seminars in Speech and Language, 8.* 101–106.

DeCurtis, M., McIntosh, N., Ventura, V., and Brooke, O. (1986). Effect of nonnutritive sucking on nutrient retention in preterm infants. *Journal of Pediatrics, 109,* 888–890.

Discippio, W., & Kaslon, K. (1982). Conditioned dysphgia in cleft palate children after pharyngeal flap surgery. *Psycho Medicine, 44, 247.*

Ernst, J. (1989). Lack of improved growth outcome related to nonnutritive sucking in very low birth weight premature infants fed a controlled nutrient intake: A randomized prospective study. *Pediatrics (83),* 706–716.

Fajardo, B., Browning, M., Fisher, D., and Paton, J. (1990). Effect of nursery environment on state regulation in very-low birth weight infants. *Infant Behavior and Development, 13,* 287–303.

Field, T., Ignatoff, E., Stringer, S., Bremman, J., Greenberg, R., Widmayer, S., & Anderson, G. (1982). Non-nutritive sucking during tube feedings: Effects on preterm neonates in an intensive care unit. *Pediatrics, 70,* 381–384.

Fielder, A. (1993). Health of children born prematurely. New treatment reduces risk of blindness. *British Medical Journal, 307,* 502.

Finlayson, M., & Garner, S. (1994). *Brain injury rehabilitation: Clinical considerations.* Baltimore, MD: Williams & Wilkins.

Fisher, S., Painter, M., & Milmore, G. (1993). Swallowing disorders in infancy. *Pediatric Clinics of North America, 28*(4), 845–853.

Gale, S. (2000). Bottle-feeding premature infants. *Advance for Speech Language Pathologists & Audiologists, 8*(10), 11–13.

Glass, G. (1968). *Introduction to gasrointestinal physiology.* Englewood Cliffs, NJ: Prentice Hall.

Goldson, E. (1987). Nonnutritive sucking in the sick infant. *Journal of Perinatology, 8,* 30–34.

Gomella, T., Cunningham, D., & Eyal, F. (1994). *Neonatology: Management, procedures, on-call problems, diseases and drugs* (3rd ed.). Stamford, CT: Appleton & Lange.

Hack, M., Estabrook, M., & Robertson, S. (1985). Development of sucking rhythm in preterm infants. *Early Human Development, 11,* 133–140.

Hamlet, S., Penny, D., & Formolo, J. (1994). Stethoscope acoustics and cervical auscultation of swallowing. *Dysphagia, 9,* 63–68.

Harrison, H. (1983). *The premature baby book.* St. Martins Press: New York.

Horton, F. Lubchenco. L., & Gordon, H. (1952). Self-regulatory feeding in a premature nursery, *Yale Journal of Biology and Medicine, 24,* 263–272.

Ichord, R. (1994). Neurology of deglutition. In Tuchman & Walter (Eds), *Disorders of feeding and swallowing in infants and children: Pathophysiology, diagnosis, and treatment* (pp. 37–52). San Diego: Singular Publishing Group.

Illingworth, R., & Lister, J. (1964). The critical or sensitive period with special reference to certain feeding problems in infants and children. *The Journal of Pediatrics, 65,* 839–848.

Jelm, J. (1990). *Oral-motor feeding rating scale.* Tucson, AZ: Therapy Skill Builders.

Jones, K. L. (1997). *Smith's recognizable patterns of human malformation.* Philadelphia, PA: W.B. Saunders Company.

Kamhi, A. (1999). To use or not to use: Factors that influence the selection of new treatment approaches. *Language, Speech, and Hearing Services in the Schools, 30,* 92–97.

Kamolz, T., Brammer, T., & Pointer, R. (2000). Predictability of dysphagia after laparoscopic Nissen fundoplication. *The American Journal of Gastroenterology, 95,* 408–414.

Kanter, W. (1994). Medical progress: A decade of experience with neonatal extracorporeal membrane oxygenation. *The Journal of Pediatrics, 124,* 335–347.

Kinner, M., & Beachy, P. (1994). Nipple feeding premature infants in the neonatal intensive-care unit: Factors and decisions. *Journal of Obstetrics, Gynecology, and Neonatal Nursing, 23,* 105–12.

Klein, M., & Delaney, T. (1994). *Feeding and nutrition for the child with special needs.* Tucson, AZ: Psychological Corporation.

Kliegman, R. (1990). Neonatal necrotizing enterocolitis: Bridging the basic science with the clinical disease. *Journal of Pediatrics, 117,* 836.

Kosko, J., Moser, J., Erhart, N., & Tunkel, D. (1998). Differential diagnosis of dysphagia in children. *Otolaryngologic Clinics of North America, 31,* 435–451.

Kramer, S. (1985). Special swallowing problems in children. *Gastrointestinal Radiology, 104,* 152–162.

Kramer, S. S., & Eicher, P. M. (1993). The evaluation of pediatric feeding abnormalities. *Dysphagia, 3,* 215–224.

Lawhon, G., & Melzar, A. (1988). Developmental care of the very low birh weight infant. *Journal of Perinatal & Neonatal Nursing, 2,* 56–65.

Layton, T., & Davis-McFarland, E. (2000). Pediatric human immunodeficiency virus and acquired immunodeficiency syndrome: An overview. *Seminar in Speech & Language, 21,* 7–17.

Lefton-Greif, M. (1997). Diagnosis and management of pediatric feeding and swallowing disorders. In D. Tuchman & R. Walter (Eds.), *Disorders of feeding and swallowing in infants and children: Pathophysiology, diagnosis, and treatment* (pp. 97–114). San Diego: Singular Publishing Group.

Logan, W., & Bosma, J. (1967). Oral and pharyngeal dysphagia in infancy. *Pediatric Clinics of North America, 14,* 47–61.

Logemann, J. (1998). *Evaluation and treatment of swallowing disorders* (2nd ed.). Austin, TX: Pro-Ed.

Long, J., Philip, A., & Lucey, J. (1980a). Noise and hypoexemia in the intensive care nursery. *Pediatrics, 65,* 143–145.

Long, J., Philip, A., & Lucey, J. (1980b). Excessive handling as a cause of hypoxemia. *Pediatrics, 65,* 203–207.

Martin, R., Siner, B., Carlo, W., Lough, M., & Miller M. (1988). Effects of head position on distribution of nasal airflow in preterm infants. *Journal of Pediatrics, 112,* 99–103.

Mason, M. F. (1994). *Speech pathology for the tracheostomized and ventilator dependent patient.* Newport Beach, CA: Voicing.

Matthew, O. (1991). The science of bottle feeding. *The Journal of Pediatrics, 119,* 511–519.

McCain, J. (1995). I want to go home. *Florida Nursing, 43,* 27–28.

McKeon, R., et al. (1992). Role of delayed feeding and of feeding increments in necrotizing enterocolitis. *Journal of Pediatrics, 224,* 764.

McLone, D. (2000). Chiari malformations. *Pediatric Neurosurgery, 32,* 164.

Measel, C., & Anderson, G. (1979). Non-nutritive sucking during tube feedings: Effects upon clinical course in premature infants. *Journal of Obstetric, Gynecologic and Neonatal Nursing, 8,* 265–272.

Meer, P. (1998) Update on feeding babies solid food. *Journal of Pediatric Health Care, 12*(3), 152–153.

Merenstein, G., & Gardner, S. (1985). *Handbook of neonatal intensive care.* St. Louis, MO: Mosby.

Messner, K. (1978). Light toxicity to newborn retina. *Pediatric Research, 12,* 530.

Miller, A. (1986). Neurophysiological basis of swallowing. *Dysphagia, 1,* 91–100.

Miller, M.J., Martin, R., Carlo, W., Fouke, J., Strohl, K., & Fanaroff. (1985). Oral breathing in newborn infants. *Journal of Pediatrics, 107,* 465–469.

Moore, K. (1988). *The developing human: Clinically oriented embryology* (4th ed.). Philadelphia: W.B. Saunders.

Morris, S. (1999a). Expanding children's diets [On-line]. Available: www.newvisions.com

Morris, S. (1999b). Children with feeding tubes [On-line]. Available: www.newvisions.com

Morris, S., & Klein, M. (1987*). Pre-feeding skills. A comprehensive resource for feeding development.* Tucson, AZ: Therapy Skill Builders.

Nelson, S., Chen,E., Syniar, G., & Christoffel, K. (1997). Prevalence of symptoms of gastroesophageal reflux during infancy. A pediatric practice-based survey. Pediatric Practice Research Group. *Archives of Pediatric Adolescent Medicine, 151,* 569–572.

Ogorek, C. (1995). Gastroesophageal reflux disease. In J. Berk. (Ed.), *Bockus gastroenterology* (pp. 445–463). Philadelphia, PA: W. B. Saunders Company.

Omari, T., Miki, K., Fraser, R., Davidson G., Haslam, R., Goldsworthy, W., Bakewell, M., Kawahara, H., & Dent, J. (1995). Esophageal body and lower esophageal sphincter function in healthy premature infants. *Gastroenterology, 109,* 1757–1764.

Omim. (2000). [On-line]. Available: http://www3.ncbi.nml.nih.gov/htbin-post/Omim/getmim

Orenstein, S., Giarrusso, V., Proujansky, R., & Kocoslis, S. (1988), The Santmyer swallow: A new and useful infant reflex. *The Lancet, 1,* 345–346.

Orenstein, S., Magill, H., & Brooks, P. (1987). Thickening of infant feedings for therapy for gastroesophageal reflux. *The Journal of Pediatrics, 110,* 181–186.

Orenstein, S., & Whitington, P. (1982). Choledochal cyst resulting in congenital cirrhosis. American *Journal of the Disabled Child. 136,* 1025–1027.

Owens, R. (1984). *Language development: An introduction.* Columbus, OH: Charles E. Merrill.

Palmer, M. (1993). Identification and management of the transitional suck pattern in premature infants. *Journal of Neonatal Nursing, 7,* 66–75.

Palmer, M., & Heyman, M. (1993). Assessment and treatment of sensory- versus motor-based feeding problems in very young children. *Infants and Younge Children, 6,* 67–73.

Paludetto, R., Robertson, S., Hack, L., Shivpuri, C., & Martin, R. (1984). Transcutaneous oxygen tension during nonnutritive sucking in preterm infants. *Pediatrics, 74,* 539–542.

Parmelle, A., Wenner, W., Akiyama, Y., Schultz, M., & Stern, E. (1967). Sleep states in premature infants. *Developmental Medicine in Child Neurology, 9,* 70–77.

Perlman, A., & Christensen, J. (1997). Topography and functional anatomy of the swallowing structures. In A. Perlman & K. Schulze-Delrieu (Eds.), *Deglutition and its disorders: Anatomy, physiology, clinical diagnosis and management* (pp. 15–42). San Diego: Singular Publishing Group.

Peters, K. (1992). Does routine nursing care complicate the physiologic status of the premature neonate with respiratory distress syndrome? *Journal of Perinatal & Neonatal Nursing, 6,* 67–84.

Pickler, R., Frankel, H., Walsh, K., & Thompson, N. (1996). Effects of nonnutritive sucking on behavioral organization and feeding performance in preterm infants. *Nursing Research, 45,* 132–135

Preiksaitis, H. Mayrand, S., Robins, K., & Diamant, N. (1992). Coordination of respiration and swallowing: Effect of bolus volume in normal adults. *American Journal of Physiology, 263,* R624–R630.

Pressman, H., & Morrison, S. (1988). Dysphagia in the pediatric AIDS population. *Dysphagia, 2,* 166–169.

Richard, K. (1991). Strategies for children with cancer. *Nutrition Focus, 6,* 1–5.

Robertson, A., & Bhatia, J. (1993). Feeding premature infants. *Clinical Pediatrics, 32,* 36–44.

Rodenstein, D., Perlmutter, N., & Stanescu, D. (1985). Infants are not obligatory nasal breathers. *American Review of Respiratory Disorders, 131,* 343–347.

Rogers, B., & Campbell, J. (1993). Pediatric neurodevelopmental evaluation. In J. Arvedson & L. Brodsky (Eds.), *Pediatric swallowing and feeding: Asessment and management.* San Diego: Singular Publishing Group.

Rossi, T. (1993). Pediatric gastroenterology. In J. Arvedson & L. Brodsky (Eds.), *Pediatric swallowing and feeding: Assessment and management* (pp. 123–156). San Diego: Singular Publishing Group.

Rudolph, C. (1998, November). *Indentification and management of reflux in the neonate.* Paper presented at the Developmental Interventions in Neonatal Care Annual Convention, Chicago, IL.

Sabiston, D. (1986). Texbook of surgery (12th ed., p. 765). Philadelphia, PA: W. B. Saunders.

Schrank, W., Al-Sayed, L., Beahm, P., & Thach, B. (1998). Feeding responses to free-flow formula in term and preterm infants. *Journal of Pediatrics, 132,* 426–430.

Schuberth, L. (1994). The role of occupational therapy in diagnosis and management. In D. Tuchman & R. Walter (Eds.), *Disorders of feeding and swallowing in infants and children: Pathophysiology, diagnosis, and treatment* (pp. 115–130). San Diego, CA: Singular Publishing Group.

See, C. (1989). Gastroesophageal reflux-induced hypoxemia in infants with apparent life threatening events (ALTEs). *American Journal of Disease of Children, 143,* 951–954.

Seikel, J., King, D., & Drumright, D. (2000). *Anatomy and physiology for speech, language, and hearing* (2nd ed.). San Diego, CA: Singular Publishing Group.

Shaker, C. (1998). Nipple feeding preterm infants: An individualized, developmentally supportive approach. *Neonatal Network, 18,* 15–21.

Shivpuri, C., Martin, R., Carlo, W., & Fanaroff, A. (1983). Decreased ventilation in preterm infants during oral feeding. *Journal of Pediatrics, 103,* 285–289.

Stanczak, D., White, J., Gouview, W., Moehle, K., Daniel, M., Novack, T., & Long, C. J. (1984). Assessment of level of consciousness following severe neurological insult. A comparison of the psychometric qualities of the Glasgow Coma Scale and the Comprehensive Level of Consciousness Scale. *Journal of Neurosurgery, 60,* 955–960.

Stevenson, R., & Allaire, J. (1991). The development of normal feeding and swallowing. *Pediatric Clinics of North America, 38*(6), 1439–1453.

Teasdale, G., & Jennett, B. (1974). Assessment of coma and impaired consciousness, *Lancet, ii,* 81–84.

Thomas, K. (1989). How the NICU environment sounds to a preterm infant. *Maternal Child Nursing, 14,* 249–251.

Topf, M. (1992). Effects of personal control over hospital noise on sleep. *Research in Nursing & Health, 15,* 19–28.

Tribotti S., & Stein M. (1992). From research to clinical practice: Implementing the NIDCAP. *Neonatal Network, 11,* 35–40.

Tuchman, D., & Walter, R. (1994). *Disorders of feeding and swallowing in infants and children: Pathophysiology, diagnosis, and treatment.* San Diego: Singular Publishing Group.

UK ECMO Collaborative Trial Group. (1996). UK collaborative randomised trial of neonatal extracorporeal membrane oxygenation. *The Lancet, 348,* 75–82.

Vice, F., Bamford, O., Heinz, J., & Bosma, J. (1994, October). *Correlation of cervical auscultation with physiologic recording during suckle feeding in newborn infants.* Paper presented at the Second Workshop on Cervical Auscultation, McLean, VA.

Vice, F., Heinz, J., Giuriati, G., Hood, M., & Bosma, J. (1990). Cervical auscultation of suckle feeding in newborn infants. *Developmental Medicine and Child Neurology, 32,* 760–768.

Walter, R. (1994). Issues surrounding the development of feeding. In D. Tuchman & R. Walter (Eds.), *Disorders of feeding and swallowing in infants and children: Pathophysiology, diagnosis, and treatment* (pp. 27–36). San Diego: Singular Publishing Group.

Weber, F., Woolridge, M., & Baum, J. (1986). An ultrasonographic study of the organization of sucking and swallowing by newborn infants. *Developmental Medicine Child Neurology, 28,* 19–24.

Widstrom, A., Marchini, G., Matthiesen, A., Werner, S., Winberg, J., & Uvans-Moberg, K. (1988). Nonnutritive sucking in tube-fed preterm infants: Effects on gastric motility and gastric contents of somatostatin. *Journal of Pediatric Gastroenterology & Nutrition, 7,* 517–523.

Willging, J. (1995). Endoscopic evaluation of swallowing in children. *International Journal of Pediatric Otorhinolaryngology, 32,* 107–108.

Wolf, L., & Glass, R. (1992). *Feeding and swallowing disorders in infancy.* Tucson, AZ: Therapy Skill Builders.

Wolf, P. (1968). The serial organization of sucking in the young infant. *Pediatrics, 42,* 943–956.

Wood, N., Marlow, N., Costeloe, K., Gibson, A., & Wilkinson, A. (2000). Neurologic and developmental disability after extremely preterm birth. *The New England Journal of Medicine, 43,* 378–384.

Woodson, R., Drinkwin, J., & Hamilton, C. (1985). Effects of nonnutritive sucking on state and activity: Term-preterm comparisons. *Infant Behavior and Development, 8,* 435–441.

Woodson, R., & Hamilton, C. (1988). The effect of nonnutritive sucking on heart rate in preterm infants. *Developmental Psychobiology, 21,* 207–213.

Zalzal, G., Anon, J., & Cotton, R. (1987). Epiglottoplasty for the treatment of laryngomalacia. *Annals of Otology, Rhinology, and Laryngology, 96,* 72.

Zemlin, W. R. (1988). *Speech and hearing science: Anatomy & physiology* (3rd ed.). Englewood Cliffs, NJ: Prentice-Hall.

ANATOMICAL STRUCTURES OF INFANT FEEDING/ SWALLOWING

Oral Cavity

Lips: They form the orifice of the mouth. Important landmarks are *vermilion zone* (red transitional area from the skin to the inner mucosa), *tubercle* (small projection in the midline of the upper lip), *philtrum* (vertical groove below the nose), and *columella* (vertical grooves that lie on either side of the philtrum). The inner surfaces of the lips are connected to the alveolar process of the *maxilla* by the *superior labial frenulum* (upper lip) and connected to the alveolar process of the *mandible* by the *inferior labial frenulum* (lower lip).

Mandible: Because of its relationship to the tongue, mandibular movement causes the tongue to raise and lower during sucking and mastication. Mandibular movements also affect lip posture, tongue position, alter the dimensions of the pharynx, and can help depress the larynx. The mandible is raised by three muscles: masseter, temporalis, and internal pterygoid. The mandible is lowered by five muscles: external pyterygoid, genio-hyoid, digastricus (anterior belly), mylo-hyoid, and genioglossus. These muscles also are responsible for lateralizing, protruding, and retracting the mandible.

Floor of Mouth: Formed by the mylohyoid muscle.

Cheeks: Also called "buccae." Serve as the lateral borders of the oral cavity and provide stability to redirect food between the molars during mastication. The cheeks are composed of muscles and subcutaneous fat. In infants, the *fat pads* or *sucking pads* are prominent and assist in reducing the size of the oral cavity. This is important for creating negative pressure during bottle or breast feeding. Sucking pads may also help prevent the cheeks from drawing in between the gums during sucking.

Tongue: The dorsum of the tongue can be anatomically divided into five sections: tip (anterior end nearest the *teeth*), blade (below the alveolar ridge), front (the area below the *hard palate*), back (the area below the soft palate), and base (area below the uvula to the *epiglottis*). The *lingual frenulum* or *frenum* begins at the floor of the mouth and extends to the midline of the underside of the tongue. In some infants, the frenum extends to the tongue tip, which can initally interfere with protrusion. The frenum stretches with age and rarely causes feeding problems.

Faucial Pillars: The *anterior faucial pillars*, or *platoglossal arch*, are the first and strongest site of sensory stimulation of the swallowing response in older children and adults. Behind them lie the *palatine tonsils* and *posterior faucial pillars* (*palatopharyngeal arches*). In children, the palatine tonsils are large and in severe cases can obstruct the opening to the *pharynx*, which may cause feeding problems.

Lateral Sulci: Spaces between the *teeth*, *mandible*, or *maxilla*. Also known as *buc-cae cavities*, these spaces are a recess where food can become lodged and cause feeding problems.

Teeth: Starting from the upper and lower front teeth and progressing backward, the *lower and upper central incisors* typically erupt between 6–10 months of age. The *lateral incisors*, *canines*, and first molars erupt between 10–20 months, followed by second molars at 20–24months. The eruption of *deciduous* dentition is useful, but not necessary, in the transition to solid foods. The loss of deciduous teeth begin between ages 6–7 years and end around 10–13 years. They are replaced with 32 permanent teeth; a process that continues until the wisdom teeth (upper and lower third molars) erupt between ages 17–21 years.

Pharynx

The pharynx of a newborn infant is only about 4 cm long. It extends from the base of the skull to the level of the fifth or lower level of the 6th cervical vertebra. This position is at about the same level as in an adult, because the lengthening of the pharynx parallels the expansion of the vertebral column. The pharynx can be divided into three sections, described below.

Nasopharynx: Extends from the base of the skull to the level of the soft palate. This area of the pharynx is made up of four muscle bundles of the superior constrictor muscle. In addition to acting as a resonator for speech, it connects the nasal cavity to the oropharynx and is a drainage area for the nose, paranasal sinuses, and Eustachian tube. Its function in swallowing is limited to closure during the swallow. If the velopharyngeal closure is not adequate, nasal regurgitation or nasal reflux can occur.

Oropharynx: Extends from the *posterior faucial arch* and *soft palate* to the level of the *epiglottis* and is composed of the two fan-shaped muscle bundles of the *middle constrictor muscle*. It includes the *valleculae*, a wedge-shaped space formed between the base of the tongue and epiglottis. The valleculae is the triggering site of the newborn infant swallow response.

Laryngopharynx: Also referred to as the *hypopharynx*, it extends from the tip of the *epiglottis* to *the cricopharyngeal segment*. This area is comprised of fibers of the *medial* and *inferior constrictor muscle* (ICM) and houses structures essential for swallowing. The bottom-most border of the ICM is made up of the *cricopharyngeus muscle* or *criocpharyngeal segment* (CP). The CP segment is the upper border of the upper esophageal segment, or lumen of the esophagus. At rest, the CP segment is tonically closed. On contraction, the CP segment opens to receive the bolus from the *oropharynx* and directs it into the *esophagus*. The *pyriform sinuses* are two anatomical "canals" through the laryngopharynx that direct food around either side of the larynx down to the CP segment. They are formed as the sides of the inferior constrictor muscles (lateral pharyngeal walls) attach to the sides of the thyroid cartilage.

Larynx

The infant larynx is relatively larger than the adult larnyx. The thyroid cartilage is broader, shorter, and lies closer to the hyoid bone. Laryngeal structures/areas involved in swallowing are the *epiglottis, aeryepiglottic folds, laryngeal vestibule, true and false vocal folds,* and *laryngeal ventricle*. During the swallow, the larynx is elevated by suprahyoid muscles. Laryngeal elevation is essential for adequate laryngeal closure during the swallow to prevent aspiration. Closure of the larynx proceeds from bottom to top, with closure of the true vocal folds, false vocal folds, and finally closure of the epiglottis over the *laryngeal vestibule*. The larynx descends in the neck with age along with the tongue.

Epiglottis: The uppermost cartilage of the larynx. At rest, the upper border of the epiglottis in infants lies at the level of the second or third cervical vertebra and elevates to the level of the first cervical vertebra during the swallow. Because of its position in the neck and its large shape, which is similar to the Greek letter omega, the tip of the infant epiglottis makes contact with the soft palate for the first 6 months of life. The *aeryepiglottic folds*, extending from the sides of the epiglottis to the arytenoid cartilages, contain the *aeryepiglottic muscle* that helps pull the epiglottis down during the swallow. Closure is also mediated by the downward pressure of the bolus and the posterior movement of the *base of the tongue*.

Laryngeal Vestibule: The opening of the larynx from the laryngeal side of the epiglottis to the level of the false vocal folds. Food that enters the vestibule during swallowing can either clear with the swallow (*vestibular penetration*) or remain (*vestibular aspiration*).

Laryngeal Ventricle: The space between the true and false vocal folds.

Esophagus

The esophagus is a flaccid, collapsed tube made up of circular (inner) and longitudinal (outer) muscle layers. Its length in a newborn infant is approximately 8–10 cm. At the top is the *upper esophageal segment*, which contains the cricopharyngeus muscle. At the bottom is the *lower esophageal segment* or *cardiac sphinctor*. When it contracts, it pushes food toward the stomach in a wave-like progression called "primary peristalsis." The radiologist will refer to the esophagus in three segments. The *cervical esophagus* runs from the suprasternal notch to the thoracic inlet. The *thoracic esophagus* runs from the inlet, around the aortic notch, to the level of the 8th thoracic vertebra. The *abdominal esophagus* contains the LES. There are three esophageal layers: epithelium, laminae propria, and muscularic mucosae. Esophageal motility problems, strictures (narrowing), and reflux (anterior return of the bolus into the esophagus and/or pharynx) are some of the common esophageal disorders in children with feeding problems.

Trachea

In infants, the trachea is about 4.0 cm long. It is short, narrow, and relatively smaller than the larynx. The tracheal cartilages are separated by ligaments. In infants, these cartilages are much closer together and very elastic (i.e., easily externally compressed). The infant trachea begins at the level of the 6th cervical vertebra. This position remains the same as the child grows because it parallels the growth of the vertebral column and descent of the larynx.

Sources: Compiled from Arvedson, J. C., & Brodsky, L. (1993). *Pediatric swallowing and feeding: Assessment and management*. San Diego: Singular Publishing Group.

Crelin, E. (1973). *Functional anatomy of the newborn*. London: Yale University Press.

Zemlin, W. R. (1988). *Speech and hearing science: Anatomy & physiology* (3rd ed.). Englewood Cliffs, NJ: Prentice-Hall.

APPENDIX

DEVELOPMENTAL COGNITIVE-SOCIAL-COMMUNICATIVE-SENSORY MILESTONES

• •

215

Age (Months)	Cognition	Socialization/Feeding	Communication	Sensory
Newborn	• Sees best at 7.5 inches • Brightness and color are enhanced • Turns head to move with object • Prefer sharp, visual contrasts • 5–8 feedings per day • Volume, pitch, and duration of sound are enhanced • Slight hearing loss until middle ear clears • Aware that sound is coming from different sources • Prefers human voice • Makes basic distinctions in vision, hearing, smell, taste, touch, temperature, and perception of pain • Filters out stimuli • Sleeps 20 hours per day	• Nipple fed, identifies nipple • Relaxed by human voice when feeding • When awake, is usually eating • Smiles automatically • Hand to mouth	• Cries to communicate needs • Speech-like sounds can be heard when feeding • Asocial	• Touch cheek, will turn in direction of hand • Wet diaper—uncomfortable • Mother's hand—comforting • Touch sensations important as source of emotional satisfaction
1	• Cries when troubled • Attracted by visual patterns • Visual memory is 2.5 sec. • Regular feedings become expected • Simple reflex activity such as grasping, sucking	• Maintains eye contact with feeder • Prefers being held • Impulsive smile	• Moves when hears human voice • Cries to gain attention • Sounds originate in throat • Happy, cooing sounds are heard	
2	• Chooses faces over objects • Reflexive behaviors occur in repetition such as opening and closing fingers • Performs repeated, circular actions with own hands • Objects evoke noticeable enthusiasm • Color perception • Simple associations emerge • Control of eye muscles • Lifts head when on stomach	• Positive response to seeing bottle • Smiles at a face • Soothed by rocking and NNS • Prefer tactile stimulation • Visually fixates on a face • Starts to put hand to bottle during feeding	• Discriminates different speech sounds • Cooing emerges from the throat • Crying continues to be main mode of communication • Delight and distress is apparent • Appearance of vowel-like noises	
3	• Able to completely focus visually • Moves eyes in search of sound source • Visual and oral exploration • Exploratory play emerges • Smiles in response to own image • Halts activity in response to hearing parent's voice	• Social skills emerge • Aware of difference between people and objects • Identification of mother • Smiles voluntarily • Does not awake as often in the night for feeding	• Produces many different noises, laugh emerges from back of throat • Produces consonant/vowel syllable • Head movement and vocalizations in response to other's speech • Speech consists mostly of vowels	

Age (months)				
4	• Localizes sounds • After object is dropped, focuses on area it came from • Control of head and arm movements, grasping • Visual memory 5–7 seconds • Senses unfamiliar places • Rolls over • Distinguishes between familiar people and strangers • Identifies mother among a gathering of people	• Spoon feeding of thin pureed consistencies introduced • May stop feeding and turn attention toward a person entering or exiting a room • Smiles at other babies • Prepares for being lifted by someone else • Enjoys being cuddled • Prefers faces and distinguishes between different faces • Laugh emerges	• Babbles most vowels and about half of the consonants • Variety of pitch in voice • Imitates people's tone of voice • Smiles directed toward speaker • Expects feeding, dressing, and bathing	• Big movements start (e.g., banging spoon on table) • Touches/looks at own hands • Brings hands together in front of body so they touch • Begins to enjoy being held up, rocked, swung, turned over, and moved
5	• Play emerges • Recognizes objects and visually follows them until out of visual field • 3–5 feedings per day • Knows there is a whole to a single part • Visual memory improves to 3 hours • Oral and tactile exploration of objects • Recalls own recent actions	• Cup drinking introduced (4–6 months) • Puts both hands on bottle • Responds accordingly to smiling or scolding • Differentiates immediate family members from other people • Imitates movements	• Talks to toys • Responds appropriately to different voices (happy, angry) • Visually fixates at a mouth • Imitates sounds and tries producing new ones • Reacts to hearing own name • Produces sounds and smiles at own image • The sounds /m/ and /b/ start to be produced	
6	• Coordinated vision and grasping of objects • Begins to perform actions on objects • Reaches to retrieve objects that have fallen • Interested in environmental consequences of their movements (cause and effect)	• Accepts semisolids from spoon with lip closure around spoon • Will "lick" or "mouth" cracker • Immature munching (up/down) chewing movements of jaw • Sucks liquids from spouted cup	• Vocalization with intonation • Communicates emotional state by vocalizing • Audible noises when excited • Exploration of mouth shape to produce new sounds • Responds to human voices without visual cues by turning head and eyes	• Increasing awareness about space • Can use thumb and fore-finger in scissors action
7	• Begins to search for toy that is out of visual field • Control of trunk and hands • Imitates actions • Sits without support • Begins to understand properties of objects (may sort by size) • Hiding games further improve visual memory • Crawls	• Rotary chew begins (lateral and vertical rotations of the jaw) • Begins to tease • Mealtime is playtime • Tries to take spoon from feeder • Begins to participate in social routines of mealtime	• Vocalizes during play • Longer utterances • Listens to others speak • Recognizes different tones in voices	
8	• Recognizes difference between color and form • Prefers complex toys • Explores properties of objects	• Shouts to gain attention • Mealtimes are "noisy" • Manipulates utensils (bangs spoons, grabs cup) • Watches others eat	• Chooses what and what not to listen to • Recognizes familiar words in context • Repeats stressed syllable • Imitates gestures • Begins to echo vocalizations • Imitates increased number of sounds	

(continued)

Age (Months)	Cognition	Socialization/Feeding	Communication	Sensory
9	• Imitates finding an object • Responses become coordinated into more complex sequences • Awaits the consequence of an action and the return of a person • Actions take on an "intentional" quality	• Can self-feed small pieces crackers • Can bring cup to mouth with two hands, holds briefly • Grabs spoon from feeder and "assists" in bringing to mouth • Prefers games consisting of action • Imitates play	• Distinguishes patterns of intonation apparent in speech • Imitates nonspeech sounds made by speaker • Gestures made socially • Jargon • May respond to some words • Listens to conversations • The words "mama" and "dada" may emerge	
10	• Identifies body parts by pointing to them • Learns from trial and error • Spontaneously searches for object in a familiar context • Depth perception emerges	• Self-feeding preferred • Helps to dress self • Expresses emotional state	• Speech sounds mirror adult sounds • Variagated babbling of consonant/vowel & CVC syllables • Follows simple commands • Combines gestures with words • Waves bye-bye • Understands "no"	
11	• Increases imitation • Identifies an object by it's properties • Creeps	• Seeks approval • Protests food dislikes • Pincer grasp developed for finger feeding	• Imitates sounds, facial expressions, actions, and rhythms • Language comprehension occurs by hearing objects labeled in familiar contexts • Approximates meaningful single words	
12	• Reaches without looking • Uses simple objects • Focuses on place object was previously in • Imitates a person who is not present • Control of legs and feet • Stands • Apposition of thumb and fore-finger	• Self-feeds with bottle • Expresses anger, affection, fear of strangers, and curiosity • Plays pat-a-cake • Gives and takes objects • Is aware of the social value of speech	• Recognizes when own name is being used • Understands simple instructions, especially if vocal or physical cues are given • Practices inflection • Understands "no" • First word may emerge • Uses one or more words with meaning • Sentence-like intonation	• Begins to tell roughly where he/she is touched • Touch sensation makes it feel good to hold things • Sensations from skin tell where body begins and ends • Sensations from own body make child feel secure and confident
13	• Learns objects have function by observing adults use them • Symbolic play with toy telephone		• Only fragments of words may be used • Use of gestures to compensate for words not saying yet	
14	• Creates means to goals • Discovery of new ways to produce the same consequence or obtain the same goal (pulls a pillow toward himself/herself in an attempt to get a toy resting on it)	• Imitates novel movements	• Enjoys rhyming songs • Uses gestures to demonstrate needs • Initiates actions with caregiver	

15–16

- Simple motor acts are imitated
- Creeps up stairs
- Walks (10–20 min.)
- Makes lines on paper with crayon

- Very upset when separated from mother
- Fear of bath
- Enjoys dancing
- Uses gross motor skills to play with toys
- Dependent behavior
- Plays alone
- Make-believe play begins

- Points to objects named
- Conversation emerges with the use of words and jargon
- Has 4–6 word vocabulary
- Comprehends names of major body parts
- Feeds himself/herself
- May have 6–7 word vocabulary
- Enjoys word games
- Uses adults for obtaining objects
- Comprehends about 50 words

17–24

- Identifies pictures
- Knows where certain objects in household are kept
- Assigns a different function to everyday objects in play
- May understand the concept of "now"
- Does not realize the consequences of his/her actions (touching a hot stove)
- Improved ability to recall objects or people without visual or tactile cues
- Identifies shapes
- Visual and auditory observations become fine-tuned
- Interest in books grows, begins to turn pages
- Accurate associations are made as a result of improved memory
- Identifies that a picture is upside down
- Attention span is short
- Comprehends "one," "many," "soon," and "after"
- May not comprehend days or time
- Gross motor skills improve
- Sleeps 12 hours per night with 1–2 hour naps

- Temper tantrums
- Resentment of new baby
- Does opposite of what told to do
- Increased interaction with others, parallel play emerges
- Still prefers solitary play
- Pretends to feed doll
- Enjoys giving others hugs
- Enjoys toys such as dolls and trucks
- Begins to role play
- Prefers toys with a lot of action
- Begins to command others
- Communicates wishes and interests
- Pretends that toys have life-like qualities

- Words are used to explain needs
- Enjoys picture books
- May comprehend more words than they can say
- Vocabulary of more than 200 words by 24 months (mostly nouns)
- Focuses on words that relate to daily life
- Combines two words
- Uses own name when talking about self
- Sings and hums
- Question asking begins
- Uses "no" often
- Realizes everything is called by a name
- Enjoys games using rhyme
- Uses physical contact to get someone's attention
- Comprehends a few personal pronouns and uses "I" and "mine"
- Mostly uses words to express feelings, but may still count on facial expression or yelling
- Uses short sentences with emerging grammar that are often not complete
- Approximately two thirds of what child says should be intelligible
- Rhythm and fluency often poor
- Volume and pitch of voice are not yet well controlled
- May take the lead in a conversation

(continued)

Age (Months)	Cognition	Socialization/Feeding	Communication	Sensory
25–29	• Begins to solve problems internally • May understand number/order concepts • Classification comprehension emerge • Walks well, goes up and down stairs alone • Uses spoon and fork • Attempts to dress self	• Dependent on adult guidance • Continues to play with dolls • Socially very immature, little concept of others as "people" • Dependent, clinging • Possessive about toys • Resists parental demands • Rigid insistence on sameness of routine • Inability to make decisions • Fear of separation • Plays tricks on people • Differentiates facial expressions of anger, sorrow, and joy	• Vocabulary grows quickly • 3–4 word sentences • "Why?" questions emerge • Focuses attention on what someone is saying to him/her	
30–36	• Understands relationship between objects • Sorting shapes and colors • Inability to take different views when reasoning • Enjoys reading and writing • May know age, but has no concept of time	• Takes turns • Enjoys brief group activities requiring no skill • Parallel play • Likes to share, uses "we" • 36 months = cooperative play • Affectionate toward parents	• May follow simple 2 and 3 step directions • Understands stories and can recall concepts in books • Uses pronouns *I, you, me* correctly • May correctly identify colors • Has about 900–1000 words • About 90% of what child says should be intelligible • Verbs begin to predominate • Explores world with language • Relates experiences so that they can be followed with reason • Should be able to give gender, name, and age	• Three to 7 years old is a critical period for sensory integration • Brain is most receptive to sensations and most able to organize them

Source: Adapted from Arvdeson & Brodsky (1993); Klein & Delaney (1994); Owens (1984); and Wolf & Glass (1992).

INDEX